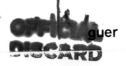

The SCIENTIFIC AMERICAN HEALTHY AGING BRAIN

Previous Books in the *Scientific American* Brain Series

The Scientific American *Book of Love, Sex, and the Brain*

The Scientific American *Brave New Brain*

The Scientific American *Day in the Life of Your Brain*

SCIENTIFIC
AMERICAN™

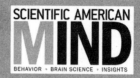

The SCIENTIFIC AMERICAN
HEALTHY AGING BRAIN

The Neuroscience of Making the Most of Your Mature Mind

Judith Horstman

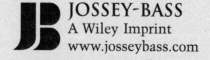

JOSSEY-BASS
A Wiley Imprint
www.josseybass.com

Published by Jossey-Bass
A Wiley Imprint
One Montgomery Street, Suite 1200, San Francisco, CA 94104-4594—www.josseybass.com

Front cover artwork © Photolibrary.

The contents of this work are intended to further general scientific research, understanding, and discussion only and are not intended and should not be relied upon as recommending or promoting a specific method, diagnosis, or treatment by physicians for any particular patient. The publisher and the author make no representations or warranties with respect to the accuracy or completeness of the contents of this work and specifically disclaim all warranties, including without limitation any implied warranties of fitness for a particular purpose. In view of ongoing research, equipment modifications, changes in governmental regulations, and the constant flow of information relating to the use of medicines, equipment, and devices, the reader is urged to review and evaluate the information provided in the package insert or instructions for each medicine, equipment, or device for, among other things, any changes in the instructions or indication of usage and for added warnings and precautions. Readers should consult with a specialist where appropriate. The fact that an organization or Web site is referred to in this work as a citation and/or a potential source of further information does not mean that the author or the publisher endorses the information that the organization or Web site may provide or recommendations it may make. Further, readers should be aware that Internet Web sites listed in this work may have changed or disappeared between when this work was written and when it is read. No warranty may be created or extended by any promotional statements for this work. Neither the publisher nor the author shall be liable for any damages arising herefrom.

Jossey-Bass books and products are available through most bookstores. To contact Jossey-Bass directly call our Customer Care Department within the U.S. at 800-956-7739, outside the U.S. at 317-572-3986, or fax 317-572-4002.

Wiley publishes in a variety of print and electronic formats and by print-on-demand. Some material included with standard print versions of this book may not be included in e-books or in print-on-demand. If this book refers to media such as a CD or DVD that is not included in the version you purchased, you may download this material at **http://booksupport.wiley.com**. For more information about Wiley products, visit **www.wiley.com**.

Library of Congress Cataloging-in-Publication Data
Horstman, Judith.
   The Scientific American healthy aging brain : the neuroscience of making the most of your mature mind / Judith Horstman. – 1st ed.
       p. cm.
   Includes bibliographical references and index.
   ISBN 978-0-470-64773-8 (cloth); ISBN 978-1-118-22087-0 (ebk.); ISBN 978-1-118-23464-8 (ebk.); ISBN 978-1-118-25915-3 (ebk.)
   1. Brain–Psychophysiology. 2. Brain–Aging. 3. Neurosciences. I. Scientific American. II. Title.
   QP376.H7554 2012
   612.8′2–dc23

                                                                                        2012001580

Printed in the United States of America
FIRST EDITION
HB Printing   10 9 8 7 6 5 4 3 2 1

CONTENTS

Acknowledgments   *xi*

Preface: Live Long, and Live Well   *xiii*

Introduction: Welcome to the New Old Age   1

What's Old, Anyway?   2

How Scientists Are Researching Your Brain   3

PART ONE How Your Brain Grows   7

Chapter 1. The Well-Aged Brain: Older and Happier   9

The Myth of a Sad Old Age   10

Actually, It's Getting Better All the Time   12

Great Late Achievers   14

Are Grandparents Safer Drivers?   16

Do You Think I'm Sexy? Apparently, Yes—at Any Age   16

A Swell of Centenarians: One Hundred Reasons to Take Care of Your Brain   20

Chapter 2. How Your Brain Grows: Zero to Sixty   21

In the Beginning: Your Fetal and Baby Brain   23

A Brief Tour of Your Brain   24

The Gray and the White: Neurons and Myelin   26

Childhood: Building the Brain   28

The Teen Brain: Not Yet Ready for Prime Time   29

Get Smart Younger, Delay Dementia Older   32

The Peak Years: Twenties to Sixties   33

Chapter 3. Your Brain Growing Older: What to Expect in a Healthy Aging Brain   3̄7̄

The Usual Effects of Aging   39

Do the Brains of Men and Women Age Differently?   40

How Memory Works: The Short Version   41

Why White Matter Matters   45

The Aging Brain: Is It Less Connected?   46

Forgetting May Be Vital to Remembering   47

Five Things Most People Get Wrong About Memory   48

The Good News: Slower Is Sometimes Better   51

More Easily Distracted: Why Multitasking Is a Task   55

PART TWO Threats to Your Brain   59

Chapter 4. What Can Go Wrong   61

When Your Brain Needs Help: How Can You Tell?   64

The Darkness of Dementia   67

Mild Cognitive Impairment: A Subtle Loss   69

Stroke: The Brain Attack   70

A Healing Stroke   72

Parkinson's Disease   74

Your Brain on Diabetes: Not So Sweet   75

Traumatic Brain Injury: A Blow to Your Thinking Brain   77

Depression: An Abnormal State   78

The Legacy of Cancer: "Chemo Brain"   81

Too Much of a Good Thing: When Medications Mess Up
    Your Mind   82

What—Me Worry?   85

Chapter 5. Alzheimer's Disease: The Brain Killer   8̄7̄

What Is Alzheimer's Disease?   88

Chasing the Cause   91

Anxiety and Alzheimer's Disease: Another Reason to
   Chill   94

Maybe It's Bad Neural Housekeeping?   97

The Search for a Cure—or Even a Treatment That Works   100

Looking Beyond the Brain   104

An Ounce of Prevention: Marijuana Might Benefit Aging
   Brains   106

The Future—Without Alzheimer's Disease   109

PART THREE How to Optimize Your Aging Brain   111

Chapter 6. The Big Five for Optimal Brain Function   113

The Cognitive Shop   116

How to Keep Your Brain Healthy and Nimble   119

Chapter 7. Exercise Your Body: Move Your Body for a Better Brain   123

This Brain Was Made for Walking   126

It's Never Too Late to Start Exercising   127

A Fine Balance: Yoga, Tai Chi, and Fall Prevention   131

Chapter 8. Challenge Your Brain   135

Educated Brains Stay Better Longer   137

Why Testing Boosts Learning   138

Do Brain Fitness Products Work?   139

Computer Training May Keep You Driving Longer   143

The Bottom Line   144

Chapter 9. Nutrition: Fuel for Thought   147

Glucose Is Not So Sweet to the Brain   151

Forget the Fructose   152

Omega-3, the Essential Oil   154

Your Brain on Berries, Chocolate, and Wine: The Flavonoid
   Connection   155

Caffeine: A Perk for Your Brain   162
Is There a Pill for That? Supplements and Vitamins   163

Chapter 10. The Social Treatment   167
You've Got a Friend, We Hope   169
Talk to Teens, Live Longer   171
Finding and Making Friends in Later Life   173

Chapter 11. Creativity, Spirit, and Attitude: Enrich Thyself   175
The Art of an Active Brain   176
Live Larger to Live Better   178
The Power of Meditation for the Aging Brain   178
Smile! It Could Make You Happier   181
Attitudes Matter: The Optimism Factor   182

PART FOUR The Future for Your Brain   185
Chapter 12. Predictions, Promises, and Possibilities   187
A Fix to Reverse Memory Decline   190
Are You Saving for Those Final Years?   191
RX for This Good Life   193

Chapter 13. Living in the Now   195
Living with an Aging Brain   196
How We (Eventually) Die   197
Going Out with a Bang: The Brain Surges Just Before Death   199
Living in the Now   200

Sources   203
Illustration Credits   219
Glossary   221
Resources for Aging and Coping   231
About the Author   235
Index   237

To all who went there before us,
and showed us the way
to age well

ACKNOWLEDGMENTS

A bit more than four years ago, I received an e-mail from Alan Rinzler, an eminent editor I knew by reputation but had never met, asking if I'd be interested in writing a book in collaboration with *Scientific American* about a day in the life of your brain. That was the beginning of what would turn out to be a challenging series of four brain books in four years. He edited three and set the tone for this one before retiring from Jossey-Bass last year. Thank you, Alan. And here's to all of those at Jossey-Bass and John Wiley & Sons who made these books possible, most of whom have worked with me on all four books: Paul Foster, who started it all with an idea about a day in the life of your brain; my editors, Nana Twumasi and Marjorie McAneny, who proffered calming support as well as edits; Carol Hartland, the production genius who pulled it all together; Bev Miller, an extraordinarily insightful copyeditor; Paula Goldstein, the terrific book designer; and the marketing crew who put my books in your hands, including Jennifer Wenzel, Samantha Rubenstein, and Jeff Puda.

Kelly A. Dakin has been of inestimable help with research and fact checks through all four books as she earned her Harvard doctorate in neurobiology. Brianna Smith, an amazing research assistant, trolled years of *Scientific American* articles—speaking of which, thanks to Karin Tucker and Diane McGarvey of *Scientific American* for their patience in finding and approving the use of hundreds of articles. And many thanks to literary agent Andrea Hurst, the godmother of the brain books who first suggested my name to Alan.

Many distinguished scientists have given me their time, expertise, and support, for which I am so very grateful. Two in particular have helped with all four of these books, reading, correcting my errors, and suggesting edits: John Dowling of Harvard College, the Llura and Gordon Gund Professor of Neuroscience, who also generously provided the basic information on brain development in this book; and R. Douglas Fields, chief of the Nervous System Development and Plasticity Section, National Institutes of Health, and editor in chief of the journal *Neuron Glia Biology*, who is as extraordinary a writer as he is a scientist. All errors are mine.

Every writer needs first readers—those who ask, "Say *what*?" or gently point out a mistake, and again I have been blessed. Ann Crew has previewed all of my books; thanks this time also to JT Long, Robin MacDonald, Ferris Urbanowski, Frank Urbanowski, Judith Auberjonois, and Joan Aragone. The very generous Sacramento Writers Who Wine have buoyed me over many rough spots.

And thanks most especially to my brilliant daughters who observed how very hard I had to work to understand neuroscience and who concluded with satisfaction that the process just might have prompted enough new neurons to see me through old age. Alcina and Ariadne, you are truly my best work.

Most of us would agree we are happier being older. As they say, it's better than the alternative. If only we didn't have to endure all the physical issues that go along with aging.

The aversion to aging has created a multibillion-dollar-a-year anti-aging industry (estimated to be $291 billion by 2015), supported by those who believe they can turn back the clock on body and mind. Alas, it's just not so. We age at different rates, and some of us may look, feel, and act younger than our age—and, yes, some healthy choices may actually keep us younger in mind and body.

But there is no such thing as anti-aging, and aging is not a disease: it's what happens if you are lucky enough to live long enough.

So here's a spoiler alert about this book. It is not about anti-aging. It's about how and why your brain grows older; the normal changes to expect in a healthy aging brain; some conditions and diseases that may challenge you and your brain, including Alzheimer's disease and other dementias; and what neuroscience is showing you can do to optimize healthy aging.

For if you can't thwart aging, there is plenty you can do to age well. Research shows, for openers, that your brain most likely will not deteriorate rapidly with age but rather will recede more subtly. Alzheimer's disease is terrible and affects millions, but it is not inevitable. Indeed, some healthful and commonsense practices are connected with lower risks of dementia.

For most of us, older is indeed happier, and researchers are finding that happiness may be its own reward: living an active, optimistic life with many friends and lots of leisure-time activities increases not only the quality of your life but the longevity of you and your brain.

The SCIENTIFIC AMERICAN
HEALTHY AGING
BRAIN

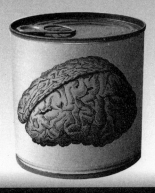

Welcome to the New Old Age

In all of history, there has never been a better time to grow old.

First, we *can* grow old. At the start of the twentieth century, the average life span was 47. Today the global average is 68, and for those born today in Western developed countries, it's around 80, nearly double in little more than a century.

The longer you live, the longer you may live. Consider this: for a 65-year-old woman today, the average—average!—life span is 84.8, or 19.8 more years. And at age 75, that jumps to 87.6 years. A man who is 75 years old today can expect to live to 85.5. If you're taking care of yourself, there could easily be more years.

Second, thanks to modern medicine and technologies, we don't look or act as old as our ancestors did. Those of us past the midcentury mark who can recall our grandparents know that with the outstanding

1

exception, they were not usually participating in an active lifestyle. If they were still alive by their 70s, often they were sedentary, ill, or failing.

True, the absolute life span has not increased, with 122 being the oldest age recorded. But more of us are living longer than at any time in the past, and living better.

What's Old, Anyway?

Today in developed countries, it seems to be accepted that young old age begins in the late 60s and that old old age comes after the age of 80.

The answer depends, of course, on who you ask. There's a remarkable generation gap when it comes to determining when old age begins according to a 2009 national survey, Growing Old in America, by the Pew Research Center. Among the nearly three thousand surveyed, those between ages 18 and 29 said they believed that the average person becomes old at age 60, middle-aged respondents put it closer to 70, and those ages 65 and above say that old begins at age 74. The researchers' conclusion after massaging the data: old age begins at 68.

But that doesn't mean you're old at 68—at least in your own mind. Other questions revealed that while young people in the survey felt their chronological age or older, oldsters don't: only 21 percent between ages 65 and 74 and 35 percent over age 75 said they feel old. In fact, a third of those aged 65 to 74 said they feel ten to nineteen years *younger* than their age, and one in six said they feel at least twenty years younger than their actual age.

There's evidence to back that up. Today's 60 and 70 year olds are to a large extent out in the workforce: 16 percent of us are still on the job (and 55 percent of those full time) because we want to be or perhaps because economics demand it. At the age that our grandparents were getting dentures and new rocking chairs (if they didn't already), we're getting braces on our teeth and investing in gym memberships, starting new businesses, trekking in Nepal, running silver marathons—and having sex: even those in their 80s report they are sexually active. And the bar has been rising. Increasingly "old old age" refers to those who have reached one hundred and up. Centenarians, in fact, are the fastest-growing demographic group in the world.

Our bodies do need more maintenance, but the specter we face and most fear is not the onslaught of bodily infirmities or even an untimely death. For most of us, it's the fear we will outlive our brain's useful life. What good are twenty extra years if our brains and minds are not able to enjoy them? If we become a burden on those we love or live out those years in institutional care?

Fortunately there's some good news about the continued health of the mature and aging brain and about how to increase your potential for an active and alert elder mind. It's going to take some work and perhaps self-discipline, two items some retirees tend to think they shed along with their jobs.

Research is showing that dementia, depression, and delusions are not normal parts of aging. Rather, they are diseases that in some cases can be averted or treated. Yes, your aging brain will slow and lose some of its edge, but it will still be able to serve you quite well. The elder brain remains plastic—able to learn new things and create new networks and memories. And the older brain is the happier brain: less prone to react in anger, more likely to recall pleasant memories than the negative past.

Indeed, there's much to enjoy in those final decades, especially if you put some effort into a healthy lifestyle, diet, and attitude.

How Scientists Are Researching Your Brain

Every day scientists are finding out more about your aging brain. This book is chock full of information from some of those research

TOOLS FOR LOOKING INSIDE YOUR BRAIN

Today's array of sophisticated technologies has come a long way since the X-ray was discovered in 1895. Here's what that alphabet soup of acronyms means:

EEG (electroencephalograph). This direct reading of the brain's electrical activity, taken from multiple electrodes placed on the scalp, is displayed as squiggly lines on a chart. It has been in use since the 1920s and is relatively inexpensive and effective. But it can't detect activity deep inside the brain very well or produce an image

CAT (computed axial tomography); also CT (computed tomography). Special X-ray equipment and computers create cross-sectional pictures of the body at different angles (*tomography* means imaging by sections). It has been used since the 1970s and has the advantage over X-rays of being able to show body sections behind other parts and in much more detail.

PET (positron emission tomography). A small amount of radioactive material is given and then detected by special cameras in images that allow researchers to observe and measure activity in different parts of the brain by monitoring blood flow and other substances such as oxygen and glucose.

MRI (magnetic resonance imaging). Magnetic fields generate a computer image of internal structures in the body. This technique is particularly good for imaging the brain and soft tissues.

fMRI (functional magnetic resonance imaging). Today's favorite, it has contributed much to our understanding. The fMRI can measure blood flow and other activity in a living, thinking brain in action and in real time, showing abnormalities, mapping functions and anatomy, and showing activity in your brain as it is happening.

MEG (magnetoencephalography). This measures the magnetic fields created by electric current flowing within neurons and detects brain activity associated with various functions in real time.

SPECT (single photon emission computed tomography). Similar to PET, it uses a small amount of radioactive tracer to measure and monitor blood flow in the brain and produce a three-dimensional image.

DTI (diffusion tensor imaging). This new technology measures the flow of water molecules along the white matter, or myelin, that makes up nearly half of your brain and connects many regions. We're just learning the importance of myelin, and this technology is not yet easily interpreted.

A word of caution: Although it is tantalizing to draw conclusions from new technologies in brain imaging, announcements about how the sources of some emotions and functions have been "mapped" in the brain need to be interpreted with care: brain-imaging technology is still very new and relatively crude, and we need to be careful about deducing cause and effect from what is now still mostly correlating observations. Although brain scans can indeed show what parts of your brain become active at certain times, scientists say they don't yet know exactly what that activity means, or even if they are seeing all the action going on. Brain researchers are still trying to figure out much of what goes on between your ears.

studies. To get all of this information, scientists use several research tools:

- *They ask you: Interviews.* Surveys and questionnaires tell us what people say they think and feel. Since the information is self-reported, it may not be completely objective. For example, recent studies where some elderly men said they have intercourse every week may not be true—but it shows these men are still thinking about sex in old age.

- *They watch you: Observation.* Watching animals and people as they react to situations, stimuli, or cognitive tests hints at what is going on in the brain and helps to connect the actions with the amount and location of brain activity.

- *They sample your tissue and fluids: Laboratory tests.* Humans and other mammals produce specific neurochemicals and hormones related to actions and emotions. Measuring these chemicals gives insights into what people are thinking and feeling, as well as what their brains are doing. For example, scientists have found that high levels of stress release chemicals that can age your brain.
- *They wire you up: Electroencephalography.* An older technique, it is still useful to record your brain's electrical activity from outside your skull.
- *They look inside your brain: Brain scans.* A host of imaging techniques and tools shows which parts of your brain are active when you are feeling or performing an activity and can show brain damage. But they have limits.

PART ONE

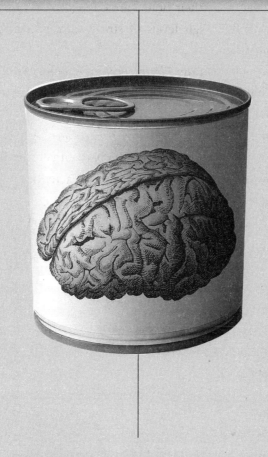

How Your Brain Grows

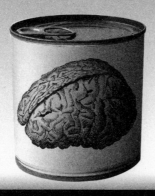

CHAPTER ONE

The Well-Aged Brain
Older and Happier

Growing older is a limiting of possibilities. At age 20, that's a depressing prospect. By age 60 or so, it's a relief. By 70 and beyond, it may be one of the reasons older folks are happier.

Yes, that's right: emotional well-being actually improves with age, according to studies from many different countries and cultures. Starting sometime after 60, folks tend to be happier, worry less, and have less stress. Wide-scale studies confirm it (and no, it's not a result of the forgetfulness of dementia).

Furthermore, research on creative accomplishments indicates that in some disciplines, such as the arts, history, and fiction writing, many people produce their best work in their 50s or even decades later. Philosophy, leadership, and politics are other areas in which the older person flourishes—hence, the term *elder statesman.*

The Myth of a Sad Old Age

Think of someone who is depressed, cantankerous, lonely, sexually inactive, and forgetful. Did an elderly person come to mind?

The answer, it turns out, depends on your age. Not surprisingly, a research team that surveyed adults at various ages found young adults (between ages 21 and 40) predicted that people would become less happy as they got older. In one survey, 65 percent of psychology students agreed that "most older people are lonely and isolated," and in another survey, 64 percent of medical students agreed that "major

---

THE MAJOR MYTHS OF AGING

There's plenty of misinformation about old age, much of it dating back to when those in their 70s and 80s were considered ancient. But quite a bit of the erroneous mythology about aging comes from media portrayals of elders. Here are a few of the myths about your brain growing older:

We Used to Think . . .	. . . But Now We Know
Older people are unhappy.	Studies show people are actually happier in their 70s than at midlife.
Depression is part of growing old.	The depression rate among healthy elders is under 5 percent—less than half the U.S. average rate of 11.26 percent (but it does increase with disability).
Retirement is terrific.	Actually, early retirement may increase the risk of death by 51 percent, and adding five years to the retirement date may lower it by 10 percent.
It's too late to improve my mind or quit bad habits.	Studies show mild cognitive impairment may be halted and perhaps reversed with exercise and other healthy activities.

depression is more prevalent among the elderly than among younger persons."

Shows how much these whippersnappers know. The truth is actually just about the opposite. Population-based surveys reveal that rates of depression are highest in those between the ages of 25 and 45, and about half as high for independently living elders.

And they are happier too. In recent studies, adults older than age 60 were actually happier than the younger respondents, and happiness continued to increase with aging. The happiest group overall is men aged 65 and older.

We Used to Think . . .	. . . But Now We Know
You can't teach an old dog new tricks.	The elder mind works differently than it did when it was younger, but it can still learn. In fact, it needs to learn new things to stay alert.
Seniors' brains are slower, and they make poor employees.	Slower perhaps—but more accurate and with better social and judgment skills than many younger workers.
Older people feel old.	A national survey shows 60 percent of those over age 65 feel ten to nineteen years younger than their chronological age.
Older people often regret their lives.	Only 1 percent of those over age 86 say their lives turned out worse than they expected.
When memory issues start, they rapidly progress to dementia.	Studies show that mild cognitive impairment doesn't always progress to dementia.
Alzheimer's disease is inevitable.	Not everyone gets dementia, and a 2011 report suggests that lifestyle changes may cut risks for some of us, perhaps as much as by half.

Where does this negative image of aging come from? Look no further than the entertainment available for your children (or grandchildren). Dubious depictions of the aged begin early in life. In Disney children's films, researchers found that 42 percent of elderly characters are portrayed in a less-than-positive light and as forgetful or crotchety. Unflattering renderings also pervade films aimed at adolescents. In a study of popular teen movies, most elderly characters were shown with negative characteristics, and a fifth fulfilled only off-putting stereotypes.

What's worse, studies show that some elderly people share these stereotypes. Talk about fiction! It might be time for a positive-aging action group.

Actually, It's Getting Better All the Time

Despite the very real and weighty concerns associated with aging, such as planning for retirement, health issues, and the death of companions and loved ones, it seems that many people in the United States actually get happier with age—and this is regardless of whether they are employed or retired, have young children at home, or live alone or with a partner. The fact is that growing older is, for many of us, growing happier.

Several studies show that happiness increases through the late 60s and into the 70s and perhaps beyond. In one study of twenty-eight thousand Americans, a third of the 88 year olds reported being "very happy," and the happiest individuals surveyed were the oldest. Indeed, the odds of being happy increased 5 percent with every decade.

Interestingly, research by Stanford University psychologist Laura Carstensen and colleagues collected over ten years found that compared with younger people, older people are more likely to recall positive than negative information, perhaps accounting partly for their often surprisingly rosy outlook on life. Older people are not generally lacking in sexual desire either. (See "Do You Think I'm Sexy?" later in this chapter.) The researchers also found that emotional experience predicted mortality: controlling for age, sex, and ethnicity, those who said they had more positive than negative emotions in everyday life not only had an improved quality of life but were more likely to have survived over a thirteen-year period.

The observation of preserved well-being flies so much in the face of stereotypes about aging that it is often met with disbelief in both the general population and the research community, Carstensen and colleagues reported. And some older people themselves share pessimistic views about the "typical" older person.

Another wide-ranging study found that in older years, the emotional flames that threatened us with self-destruction have become comforting embers in most cases. Passions run deep, but not as hot and certainly not as out of control. They reported that

- Happiness peaked around age 20—and then again in those who were in their early 70s, when their feeling of well-being was up to late-teen levels.
- The middle years may be the hardest. General well-being fell sharply through the age of 25, stress peaked between the ages of 22 and 25, worry persisted for those between their 20s and 40s—and both decreased drastically after the mid-50s.
- Anger and stress steeply declined after the early 20s.
- Sadness increased through the 40s, falling off in the mid- to late 50s.
- Oldsters recalled fewer negative memories than younger adults did, and positive emotions outweighed negative ones

The data came from a 2008 phone survey of 340,847 randomly selected adults aged 18 to 85 performed by the Gallup Organization. The researchers in the study noted that the findings fit in with proposals that "older people are more effective at regulating their emotions than younger adults" and that older adults tend to "recall fewer negative memories than younger adults" do.

These findings come from a fairly average slice of the middle-class U.S. population and are similar to studies from more than seventy countries that show a U-shaped pattern of youthful happiness followed by midlife worry and stress and then later-life happiness.

In this study, about 29 percent of those queried had a college degree and a median monthly average household income between $3,000 and $3,999. During the call, participants were asked to rate how they currently felt their life stood on a scale of 0 ("the worst possible life for you") to 10 ("the best possible life for you"). They were then asked if they had felt differently (happiness, enjoyment, stress, sadness, anger, and worry) "a lot of the day yesterday."

"As people age, they are less troubled by stress and anger," researchers noted in their study, which was led by Arthur Stone of the Department of Psychiatry and Behavioral Science at Stony Brook University. "And although worry persists, without increasing, until middle age," they continued, "it too fades after the age of 50."

This is not true for everyone, of course. Many do feel less happy with aging, including some people facing challenges with health or mobility issues, financial problems, or feelings of loneliness or loss. But quite a few of us are not just getting older; in terms of well-being, we're getting better.

Great Late Achievers

Many well-known people have produced some of their best work after their 60s, some made major accomplishments well into old old age, and some of our iconic rock and roll figures are still, well, rocking and rolling. At 69, Mick Jagger and Keith Richards (born in 1943) are still Rolling Stones; at 71, Bob Dylan remains Forever Young (1941); at 73, Tina Turner (1939) is still turning heads; and at age 86, Tony Bennett (1926) is performing and painting.

And it's not just performers: scientists have among the best of aging brains. Two of the most eminent scientists of the twentieth

AN HONOR ROLL OF GREAT OLD BRAINS

Herein is proof that life begins, or continues in fine fettle, after age 70. Just a few examples:

- At 70, Sophocles (496–406 B.C.) wrote *Electra* and *Oedipus at Colonus,* and at 83, he held office in Athens.
- At 71, Golda Meir (1898–1978) was named prime minister of Israel.
- At 75, Helen Keller's (1886–1968) book, *Teacher*, was published; Pablo Picasso (1881–1973) completed his portrait *Sylvette*, married for the second time at 77, then executed three series of drawings between ages 85 and 90.
- At 74, Giuseppi Verdi (1813–1901) wrote *Otello,* and at age 78, he wrote *Falstaff.*
- At 81, Benjamin Franklin (1706–1790) effected the compromise that led to the adoption of the U.S. Constitution, and at 82, Queen Victoria ruled England (1819–1901).
- At 86, Agatha Christie (1890–1976), who was later diagnosed with Alzheimer's disease, wrote her final mystery.
- At 88, Michelangelo (1475–1564) was painting and designing the church of Santa Maria degli Angeli e dei Martiri in Rome, and Konrad Adenauer (1949–1963) was chancellor of Germany.
- At 89, Arthur Rubinstein (1887–1982) gave one of his greatest recitals in New York's Carnegie Hall, Albert Schweitzer (1875–1965) headed a hospital in Africa, and architect Frank Lloyd Wright (1869–1959) completed New York City's Guggenheim Museum.
- At 91, Eamon de Valera (1882–1975) served as president of Ireland, Adolph Zukor, who lived to 103 (1873–1976), was chairman of Paramount Pictures, and mystery writer P. D. James (1920) published an acclaimed new book.
- At age 92, Andy Rooney (1919–2011) was commenting on television's *60 Minutes.*
- At 94, cellist Pablo Casals (1876–1973) conducted a performance and received the U.N. Peace Medal.
- At 100, Anna Mary Robertson Moses (1860–1961), who took up painting at 76, was still working as Grandma Moses.

century, Albert Einstein (1879–1955) and Thomas Alva Edison (1847–1931), worked up to the time of their deaths at ages 76 and 84, respectively. Nobel laureate Eric Kandel (1929) and neuroscientist Brenda Milner (1918), who received a major award at age 92, are among many elder scientists who have not retired.

Are Grandparents Safer Drivers?

Those added years may also add up to safety. Grandchildren seem to be 50 percent safer in crashes when driven by grandparents than by their parents, a study in *Pediatrics* finds.

Researchers looked at a cross-sectional study of motor vehicle crashes from January 15, 2003, to November 30, 2007, involving children aged 15 years or younger. The cases were culled from insurance claims with data collected by follow-up telephone surveys. They found that children driven by grandparents made up 9.5 percent of the sample but resulted in only 6.6 percent of the total injuries, even though the study also revealed the grandparents did not always use the best available child-restraint systems in the car. Researchers speculated there was an unaccounted-for protective grandparent driving style and wondered if grandparents, made nervous about the task of driving with the precious cargo of their grandchildren, establish more cautious driving habits. Of note is that these were younger grandparents for the most part, with the median age 58, although the age range went from 43 to 77.

Do You Think I'm Sexy? Apparently, Yes—at Any Age

Health willing, age does not wither sexual desire. Recent studies and surveys show the brains of those well over 60 years old want and enjoy sex.

In a national survey, more than three-quarters of men aged 75 to 85.5 and half of their female counterparts reported interest in sex and said they were sexually active. Among 75 to 85 year olds, 26 percent said they were sexually active.

Other studies find that age plays a role in marital happiness. A longitudinal study by sociologist Debra Umberson of the University of Texas at Austin and her colleagues measured the independent effect of age—as opposed to duration of marriage—and discovered that the older the spouses, the more likely they are to have a good marriage. They suggest it's perhaps because older couples are calmer and less emotionally reactive in marital conflicts than younger people or because they better appreciate their partner's positive traits.

Studies also suggest that in old age, men seem to want sex more than women do—and they get more, or at least they say they do (that doesn't seem much different than for younger men).

That could be partially explained by the dearth of men to partner aging women, who survive them. The American Association for Retired Persons (AARP) commissioned the Sex, Romance, and Relationships: 2009 AARP Survey of Midlife and Older Adults, the third it has prepared in the past decade.

The report queried about 1,670 people 45 years and older about sexual attitudes and practices and found that even in old age, men continue to think about sex more often than women do, see it as more important to their quality of life, engage in sexual activities more often, are less satisfied if they don't have a partner, and are twice as likely as women (21 percent versus 11 percent) to admit to sexual activity outside their relationship.

And, the report continues, both the frequency and satisfaction of sexual encounters were higher among those unmarried and dating (or engaged) individuals than among the married. Forty-eight percent of those who are single and dating said they have intercourse at least once a week, compared to 36 percent of those

---

FIVE GREAT THINGS ORGASM DOES
FOR YOUR AGING BRAIN

Love, the ultimate socialization, is good for us, and research also shows that sex is good for the brain in at least five ways:

1. Nourishes it. Sexual activity increases blood flow, pulse rate, and respiration. In short, it is a cardio workout that bathes your brain in oxygen.
2. Relaxes it. Relieves stress and depression, which are connected with greater dementia risks.
3. Eases pain, which contributes to stress and depression.
4. Quiets your anxiety-ridden amygdala, the part of your brain that activates the fight-or-flight response. In fact, it has to tune way down for you to have an orgasm.
5. Renews it. Orgasm may prompt the growth of new brain cells in the hippocampus of your aging brain, according to animal studies.

---

who are married. In addition, 60 percent of dating singles are satisfied with their sex lives compared to 52 percent of those who are married.

Overall, however, there has been a dip in reported satisfaction with sexual activity: in 2004, 51 percent told AARP they were satisfied with their sex lives, and in 2009 it was 43 percent. One possible factor for the cooling ardor among elders: the economic chill and concerns. The percentage who said better finances would make their sex lives more satisfying increased from 2004 to 2009 (from 17 to 26 percent among men and 9 to 14 percent among women).

Age can affect some sexual activities in men, who may have erectile dysfunction and find it more difficult to get or keep an erection, but older women don't usually have as many problems with sexual function. Of course, good health is equated with good sex, and in the AARP survey, health was among the top concerns voiced about sexual satisfaction. Women outliving their male partners and potential partners may account for their getting less sexual activity in later years, but men lose more years of sexual activity due to health issues than do women. Frailty or mobility problems can also take the bloom off sexual performance.

Sex among the aging was confirmed by another study of sex life in the United States that looked at reports from more than eight thousand people in three databases. It found that among those aged 65 to 74, 67 percent of men and 40 percent of women said they had been sexually active in the past year. Even among the oldest in the report, those 75 to 85 years old, 38.9 percent of men and 16.8 percent of women were sexually active.

And apparently still acting like crazy, irresponsible kids. One of the really startling findings shows that older is apparently not wiser: homosexual or heterosexual, the AARP study found that only one in five sexually active older singles reported using a condom regularly, and only 12 percent of the men and 32 percent of women said they used one every time. Not surprisingly, grandparents and even great grandparents had sexually transmitted diseases, from vaginitis to syphilis, gonorrhea, and genital warts, and 1 percent had HIV/AIDS. Data from the Centers of Disease Control and Prevention show that sexually transmitted diseases have skyrocketed among those 55 and older in the past few years.

One caveat: Remember that all of these studies about sexual activity depended on self-reporting—what the participants *said* about their sexual activity—and a slightly cynical person might be a wee bit suspicious at the level of activity the elderly men reported. So we might want to take the claims of men about their later life sexual activity with a grain of salt. Even so, if nothing else, these study results sure show older guys are thinking about sex quite a bit.

A Swell of Centenarians: One Hundred Reasons to Take Care of Your Brain

Jeanne Calment of France was 122 when she died in 1997, making her the longest-lived person known to date. Reaching the age of 100 years or more used to be rare. But today centenarians are the fastest-growing age group in the United States, with more than seventy-two thousand as of 2010. Experts predict there may be as many as 1 million by 2050.

If you're 60 years old (or younger) today, you could be in that group. You'll have plenty of company near your age: people aged 80 and older are the fastest-growing portion of the total population in many countries. By 2040, the number of people 65 or older worldwide will hit 1.3 billion, according to the National Institute on Aging. For the first time in human history, there will be more people in the world aged 65 and older than there will be children under the age of 5, with the most rapid increase in developing countries.

If you do live to 100, you'll want your mind intact, and if you are fortunate enough to possess a certain gene, it ups the odds of aging smartly. Nir Barzilai of the Albert Einstein College of Medicine and his colleagues examined 158 elderly people of Ashkenazi Jewish descent. Centenarians who passed a thirty-question test were two to three times as likely to have a common variant of the so-called CETP gene as those who did not, and those between ages 75 and 85 were five times as likely. The CETP gene variant leads to larger-than-normal cholesterol particles in the blood, the size perhaps making them less likely to lodge in the lining of blood vessels and thus lowering the risk of heart attack and stroke, which damage the brain.

But genes are not destiny, as studies of identical twins show. Your lifestyle practices play a major part in the health of your brain. A goodly part of this book examines normal aging, the threats to your brain health, and what you can do that could lower your risks of dementia and other brain-based conditions and perhaps join that premier One Hundred Club.

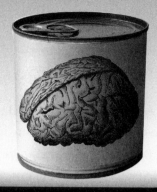

CHAPTER TWO

How Your Brain Grows
Zero to Sixty

Your brain is a work in process. From conception to death, it keeps on growing, changing, and adapting as it creates and dissolves networks and memories.

We used to think we were born with all the brain cells we'd ever have, and when they were gone, that was it. That's because your brain cells (neurons), unlike other cells in your body, can't reproduce themselves. But scientists now know that new neurons continue to arise in some parts of the brain, right up to the time of death. This is called neurogenesis.

Scientists also thought the brain was set in its ways and not able to change easily. But research has shown we are making new connections among and between brain cells all the time. Functions thought to be hardwired are turning out to be adaptable. Even as

THE FACTS ABOUT YOUR AMAZING BRAIN

- Your brain is a three-pound wonder. It occupies a scant 2 percent of your body but sucks 20 percent of your energy—enough to light a 25-watt bulb.

- Your brain fits snugly into your small skull. If its many creases, folds, and layers were spread out, it would take up more than three times that area.

- Your brain is jam-packed with functions, programs, connections, and interconnections that often overlap with other functions. It's more like a Rube Goldberg contraption than the computer to which it is so often compared. That's probably because its many complex and diverse functions have evolved over time, piggybacked onto basic functions that intertwine in ways that are still not completely understood.

- Your brain has more cells than there are stars in the Milky Way: 100 billion cells called neurons, six times that or more cells called glia, and an estimated 40 quadrillion connections. To reach those numbers, your fetal brain had to generate more than 500,000 cells per minute in the early stages of development.

- There used to be more. By the time you are born, you have lost half the neurons you had as a fetus, and in your teens, another major pruning takes place as your brain streamlines itself for optimal function.

you read this, your brain is changing in response to the very act of reading, the words you read, and the ideas the words provoke. This is neuroplasticity.

And we recently learned that genes are not destiny. Yes, your genes are set in the DNA you inherit and can't be changed, but not all of them are active, or active to the same degree. Moreover, some of them can be affected dramatically by life experiences, including what we see, do, eat, feel, and think. This is epigenetics.

This triumvirate of neurogenesis, neuroplasticity, and epigenetics is terrific news for your aging brain.

- Most of your brain cells are as old as you are and will last until you die. In contrast to other cells in your body, they do not reproduce themselves (except in select areas).

- Your brain continues to develop and mature long after birth. Some parts aren't fully developed until late adolescence, and your brain doesn't really mature until age 20 or so, after rewiring itself.

- Your brain is changing all the time. Scientists are discovering the brain makes new neurons in some areas, is constantly making and breaking networks and connections to meet new needs, and is fine-tuning gene activity—and does so into old age.

- Your brain can adapt after many (but not all) insults and injuries. In some cases, a healthy part of your brain can take over the function of a damaged area. And it grows to fit your functions. The more you repeat an action or a thought, the more brain space and connections are dedicated to it.

- Your brain never sleeps. Much as a gardener prunes away spent blooms and branches, the brain prunes itself throughout your life, cutting off less-used connections and strengthening more useful ones to create stronger neural bonds.

- In the last few minutes before death, a surge of activity has been seen in the brain. Alas, no one has yet been able to explain what that means.

In the Beginning: Your Fetal and Baby Brain

Your brain begins with one cell from each of your parents when that particular sperm and egg meet, mate, and begin the business of building you. Around the third week after conception, something called the neural plate forms along the embryonic backbone. This is the bedrock that will produce the cells that eventually make up your brain.

In the months before birth and the year that follows, your brain will grow virtually all of its hundreds of billions of cells. But your six-month-old brain is only about 30 percent of its adult size. For the next three years, it will continue to grow (though not quite so quickly) as your neurons grow and make connections, reaching its final weight when you're about 20 years old. While it is growing, it's also pruning away unneeded neurons for leaner, meaner, faster networking. Eventually as many as 70 percent of your original brain cells will be pruned and die off.

Don't worry: you have plenty left. Each of those billion or so neurons can communicate with hundreds of thousands of other neurons and can (and do) change hookups and networks all the time even into old age. Some of these will be temporary and fleeting, rather like a one-night stand, and others will become more established with repeated use, forming a lasting partnership.

A Brief Tour of Your Brain

As your brain develops from fetus to adult, it grows in much the same way it evolved over time, from the spinal cord on up. The brain sections that are oldest, such as the brain stem, mature fastest, and the newer parts, such as the thinking brain or the neocortex, mature last.

The hindbrain, sometimes referred to as the primitive brain, sits at the top of the spine and takes care of the automated basics: breathing, heartbeat, digestion, reflexive actions, sleeping, and arousal. It includes part of the spinal cord, which sends messages to and from the brain to the rest of the body; and the cerebellum, which coordinates balance and rote motions.

From here up, your brain is divided into two hemispheres connected by a thick band of fibers and nerves called the corpus callosum. Most brain parts come in pairs, one in each hemisphere. Although the halves are similar, they are not twins: each functions slightly differently from the other, communicating through the corpus callosum.

Your limbic system, or "emotional brain," is tucked deep inside the bulk of the midbrain. It acts as the gatekeeper between the spinal cord below and the cerebrum (or "thinking brain") above, regulating survival mechanisms such as sleep cycles, hunger, emotions, and, most important, fear, sensory input, and pleasure.

The ever-alert amygdala resides here, ready to sound the fight-or-flight alarm. It helps decide whether an experience is pleasurable or bad and whether it should be repeated or avoided. It sends that message along to the hypothalamus, which produces and releases chemicals that spur your body to action, and to the hippocampus, your gateway to long-term memory, which helps sort through and record memories of the event, including where and when and with whom it happened. More important, the hippocampus is one of the brain areas in humans known to make new neurons.

The so-called pleasure center, or reward circuit, is based in the limbic system, involving the nucleus accumbens, the ventral tegmental area (VTA), and the caudate nucleus—the midbrain reward and moti-vation systems that are connected with pleasure and addiction. When you are experiencing something you like very much, such as sex or music, a pathway (called the VTA-accumbens pathway) evaluates how good the experience is and sends that rating along to other parts of your reward circuit, including your amygdala and prefrontal cortex. There they file it away: the more rewarding the experience, the more likely your brain is to want to repeat it.

The thinking brain—the wrinkly and crevassed cerebrum, the part we usually see when we picture a brain—sits like a crown on the very top of your brain, covered with the nickel-thin layer of the cerebral cortex (or neocortex). This is the most recently evolved part of the brain—the part, some say, that makes us human. This is also the part that matures last in our journey from embryo to adult. Its four major lobes control thought, reasoning, language, planning, and imag-ination. The frontal lobes take care of reasoning, the occipital lobes in the back process what you see, and the temporal lobes (above your ears) are responsible for what you hear and for understanding speech and appreciating music. The parietal lobes running across the top and sides of the brain are the primary sensory areas, taking in information about taste, touch, and movement.

Eventually your thinking brain will coordinate and process all the important information it is receiving from your limbic and reward systems, including danger signals. But at first, your emotional brain is in charge. There are more connections running from your emotional to your thinking brain than the other way around, so your emotional brain will rule at first in any tug of war between feeling and thinking, something that all of us already know.

The Gray and the White: Neurons and Myelin

Neurons—those little grey cells—are what we think of when we think of brain cells, and they are indeed crucial. They are concentrated in the top layers of the brain, where they are connected by and share information through synapses.

But they are not the only brain matter that matters. White matter, formed by specialized glial cells, makes up the other half of your brain. It's essential for efficient and effective communication among those billions of neurons, helping gray matter form circuits.

Until very recently, the importance of myelin wasn't understood: many scientists thought of it as mere insulation. It is indeed insulation, but it is much more. A white fatty substance that coats and protects individual axons—the extensions that send information out from neurons—it helps speed transmission among your neurons and various brain areas. Like the trunk lines that connect telephones in different parts of a country, this white sheathing helps connect neurons in one region of the brain with those in other regions.

It's also responsible for your maturing brain. Myelin is only partially formed at birth, expands in spurts, and gradually develops in different parts of the brain up through our 20s. The timing of this growth and degree of completion can affect learning and the development of self-control (and explains why teenagers may lack it). Faulty or missing myelin in the central nervous system can contribute to several debilitating diseases, most notably multiple sclerosis.

Myelin is laid on axons somewhat like electrical tape, wrapped up to 150 times between every neural node. Electrical signals, unable to leak out through this sheath, jump swiftly down the axon from node to node. When they are coated with myelin, nerve impulses race down axons on the order of one hundred times faster. Without myelin, the signal leaks and dissipates.

This wrapping occurs at different ages, generally proceeding in a wave from the back of the cerebral cortex (shirt collar) to our front (forehead) as we grow into adulthood. The frontal lobes are the last places where myelination occurs. These regions are responsible for higher-level reasoning, planning, and judgment—skills that come with age and experience. Researchers speculate the brain doesn't finish wrapping axons until adulthood and that skimpy forebrain myelin is one reason that teenagers don't have efficient and adult decision-making abilities.

As the brain matures from childhood to adulthood, axons continue growing, gaining new branches and trimming others in response to experience, and the precision of the connections among regions improves. Once axons are myelinated, potential changes are more limited, which explains why it can be harder, but not impossible, for older brains to learn new tricks,

Studies on animal brains show that myelin can change in response to mental experience and a creature's developmental environment. Numerous studies have confirmed that rats raised in enriched environments (those with access to abundant toys and social interaction) had more myelinated fibers in the corpus callosum—the hefty bundle of axons that connects the brain's two hemispheres. In fact, changes can be seen in white matter and in neurons in brain images after (or as) we learn new skills, ranging from playing computer games to golf, to reading, to juggling, to playing the piano.

TOO MUCH, TOO YOUNG: AUTISM AND BIG BRAINS

Children with autism often lag others of the same age in both basic and social skills, but that's apparently not due to a lack of brain cells. In fact, neuroscientists are now suspecting that excess brain growth and a failure of pruning could be a cause.

Toddlers with autism tend to have large brains for their age (known as brain overgrowth), and researchers have shown a correlation between the degree of excess growth and the severity of autism symptoms. Eric Courchesne, director of the Autism Center of Excellence at the University of California, San Diego, and his colleague, Cynthia Schumann, have published data in a recent issue of the *Journal of Neuroscience* that suggest the excess brain growth starts in the first year of life, if not sooner.

Using magnetic resonance imaging scans, the researchers found overgrowth in the brains of autistic children as young as 18 months. By age 30 months, the autistic brains were 7 percent larger on average than those of the control groups. Why exactly excessive brain growth is related to autism remains a mystery, but the study helps to confirm that signs of the disorder appear early—knowledge that could lead to detection and treatments, such as behavior therapy, at a younger age.

Childhood: Building the Brain

By early childhood, your brain has grown to 95 percent of its final size. Now it settles down to the important business of creating networks: the matrix in which information will be ordered and recorded. It is busy creating the brain that will be you.

Neuroscientists have imaged brains over the years from ages 7 to 20 to show that it organizes and reorganizes itself with more long-range connections as it matures, while short-range connections tend to get weaker over time. How well the connections are made may dictate age limits for learning new skills—windows of opportunity, or critical periods, when certain learning can occur readily.

An example: Learn a foreign language after puberty, and you are destined to speak it with an accent; learn the language as a child, and you will speak it like a native. The difference occurs because the brain circuits that detect speech rewire themselves according to the sounds we hear only as a child. It loses the connections that would allow us to hear sounds unique to foreign languages. In evolutionary terms, after childhood, the brain has no reason to retain connections to detect sounds that it has never heard. Such critical periods are also one of the main reasons adults don't recover as well from brain injuries as do children. Yet experiments suggest that myelination continues into our mid-50s and perhaps much longer, albeit on a much subtler level.

It's all part of the neuroplasticity that continues well into old age. Your brain creates and dissolves thousands of networks while you are loving, living, and experiencing life.

The Teen Brain: Not Yet Ready for Prime Time

Since decision-making areas of the human brain are still developing and it doesn't reach full development until after the early 20s, it may explain why teenagers show poor judgment in risky situations. Some of the most life-threatening risks are especially common during the teenage years.

The unfinished architecture of the developing brain, seen using magnetic resonance imaging over the past two decades, shows that the human brain undergoes major remodeling during childhood and throughout the teen years—anatomical changes that may be related to the risk taking, novelty seeking, and impulsivity that characterize teen behavior.

Looking back at our adolescence—or more disconcertingly, looking right now at our kids or grandkids—it's clear the teen brain is still a work in process. Here are some examples that show the decision-making areas of the teen brain aren't fully developed (as if we needed any):

- Both males and females between the ages of 16 and 20 are at least twice as likely to be in car accidents as drivers between the ages of 20 and 50. Auto accidents are the leading cause of death among 15 to 20 year olds, and 25 percent of young drivers killed in motor vehicle crashes in 2008 had blood alcohol levels over the legal limit.
- Three million adolescents contract sexually transmitted diseases every year. People younger than 29 accounted for 39 percent of all new HIV cases in 2009, making AIDS the tenth leading cause of death among those 15 to 24 years old.
- Addiction begins in adolescence. Forty percent of adult alcoholics report having their first drinking problems between the ages of 15 and 19, and gambling typically begins by age 12. Evidence of pathological or problem gambling is found in 10 to 14 percent of teens.

Full maturation of the brain's executive function—the processes that allow us to plan, organize, and execute complex behaviors—is still under way, along with a key contributor that helps to guide voluntary behavior: working memory, that is, the ability to temporarily hold and manipulate new information. Some research shows that teens are not as efficient in recruiting areas that support working memory. Pruning gray matter is basic for brain maturation, and so is adding more myelin, which speeds up neuronal transmissions and makes the prefrontal cortex better able to control voluntary and planned behaviors.

Evidence continues to show that risky business may be hard-wired into the adolescent brain, but not because teens fail to weigh risks against benefits; in fact, most teens do so conscientiously.

THE BRAIN CHEMICAL AND ELECTRIC

Your brain is more than geography. It's chemistry and electricity as well. The neurons that carry information throughout your body—some as long as three feet—are separated by microscopically tiny gaps called synapses. Each neuron can communicate with hundreds of thousands of other neurons by releasing neurotransmitters—chemicals to carry messages over the synaptic gap—or by a minute electrical impulse. Billions of tiny blood vessels (capillaries) feed your brain, carrying oxygen, glucose, nutrients, and hormones to brain cells so they can do their work.

There are more than one hundred different neurotransmitters. Here are some your brain uses every day:

- Acetylcholine gets us going: it excites cells, activates muscles, and is involved in wakefulness, attentiveness, anger, aggression, and sexuality. Alzheimer's disease is associated with a shortage of acetylcholine.
- Glutamate is a major excitatory neurotransmitter, dispersed widely throughout the brain. It's involved in learning and memory.
- GABA (gamma-aminobutyric acid) slows everything down and helps keep your system in balance. It helps regulates anxiety.
- Endorphins act as hormones and neurotransmitters. They reduce pain sensations and increase pleasure. (The name, by the way, is a combination of end(ogenous) (m)orphine.)
- Epinephrine (also called adrenaline) keeps you alert and your blood pressure balanced, and it jumps in when you need energy. It's produced and released by the adrenal glands in times of stress. Too much can increase anxiety or tension.
- Dopamine is vital for voluntary movement, attentiveness, motivation, and pleasure. It's a key player in addiction.
- Serotonin helps regulate body temperature, memory, emotion, sleep, appetite, and mood. Many antidepressants work by regulating it.
- Oxytocin is both a hormone and a neurotransmitter. It plays a key role in labor, breast milk production, mother love, romantic love, and trust.

However, recent studies show that teens tend to put more emphasis on the benefits rather than risks when making decisions. So after carefully considering the risks and benefits of a situation, the teenage brain all too often comes down on the side of the benefits—and chooses the risky action: more evidence that with age comes wisdom.

Get Smart Younger, Delay Dementia Older

Here's some advice for your kids and grandkids (as if they'd listen): the more education they get at a younger age, the better for their aging brains.

Research suggests that mental activity in young adulthood helps keep dementia at bay later. A team of psychologists at the University of Toronto, intrigued that highly educated adults with Alzheimer's disease seemed to cope better with brain deterioration, scanned the brains of fourteen adults ages 18 to 30 and nineteen seniors beyond age 65 as they performed various memory tests. Among the older subjects, those who had had the most years of formal education during their youth did the best.

These seniors used their frontal lobes for recall, while the top young participants primarily used their medial temporal lobes. The team concluded that age may cause trouble in recruiting the temporal lobes, so the seniors used the frontal lobes, responsible for general cognition, to help out, and apparently having pushed the brain further during their college days made that substitution more effective. Highly educated adults seemed better able to use alternative brain networks.

If you're already past the age of 30, the experts say you should start challenging yourself now (whatever age "now" might be). Learn a language or a musical instrument, take classes, play cards, start a new hobby. Just keep learning.

However, these findings don't mean that education makes you immune to dementia. Researchers have also found that once dementia symptoms emerge, the well educated lose their memory faster. Researchers have speculated that the better educated unconsciously compensate as the brain changes with age, so early symptoms of dementia don't show up as soon. By the time disease overwhelms the brain and symptoms become severe enough to lead to a diagnosis of dementia, the memory decline is more rapid because the degeneration is at a later stage.

Past studies have shown that challenging the brain with activities, such as solving puzzles, undertaking a new and challenging project, or reading books, is connected with a lower risk of dementia. But researchers do not yet know if these mental challenges truly protect the brain or if the people who engage in these activities are simply better educated and in a better socioeconomic group, thus benefiting from better nutrition and health care in general.

The Peak Years: Twenties to Sixties

The years from 20 to 60 are peak for the brain in many ways. This is the time when our brain is both physically mature and still resilient. It's when we find our life's work and loves and function at our best in body and mind.

By your 20s, your brain has reorganized its networks for better connections. Pruning and an increase in myelin have streamlined and connected your brain for optimal functioning. Life experiences will have shaped your brain through neurogenesis, neuroplasticity, and epigenetics and will keep on shaping and reshaping it.

Neurogenesis is still not well understood. There are still many questions about where new neurons arise in the adult brain and if they stick around. But it is clear that neurons are born in the adult human brain in at least two specific brain regions: the subventricular zone, after which they migrate to the olfactory bulb (involved in olfaction, of course), and the dentate gyrus, a specific area of the hippocampus.

Neurons born here appear to stay put and integrate into local circuits within the hippocampus. They seem to be activated by experiences and could very well make unique contributions to learning and memory. With neuroplasticity and new experiences, the brain forges new connections among neurons, even creating new networks to take over functions for parts of the brain that have been injured. In fact, new research is suggesting that your prefrontal cortex, which is involved with decision making, social interaction, and many other personality traits, is still changing throughout the adult years.

Since 1956, the Seattle Longitudinal Study has closely tracked the same six thousand or so adults over their life spans and discovered that mental abilities don't decline in midlife. Some skills may start to decline in young adulthood, such as memorization and perceptual speed, but verbal abilities, spatial reasoning, simple math abilities, and abstract reasoning skills all improve in middle age. In fact, the studies show that middle-aged adults performed better on four out of six cognitive tests than they did as young adults, says study leader Sherry Willis of the University of Washington in Seattle. In another study, when researchers looked at the performance of pilots and air traffic controllers ages 40 to 69, they found the middle-aged brain took longer to catch on to new tests than younger counterparts but ultimately outperformed them.

Epigenetics is another way your brain changes itself, by changing your genes—or more correctly, the activity of certain genes. Your genome—the total deoxyribonucleic acid (DNA) that you inherit from your ancestors and that contains the instructions for making your unique body and brain—doesn't change. But there is another layer of information, called the epigenome, stored in the proteins and chemicals that surround and stick to your DNA (*epi* means above or beyond). It's a kind of chemical switch or volume control that determines which genes are activated (or not): it tells your genes what to do, where, when, and how much. Researchers have discovered that the epigenome can be affected by many things, from aging and diet to environmental toxins to even what you think and feel. This means your experiences can literally change your mind by shutting down or revving up the production of proteins that affect your mental state. So your brain development is never done. Your brain will continue to change until it finally dies. It will make new connections and will also create new neurons in some regions, even into very old age and in very sick brains up until the time of death. Although we don't know yet if (or how well) these new brain cells are integrated or what role they play, the brains of terminal cancer patients, donated for research after death, showed new neuron growth to the end. Your life experiences will also shape and refine your physical brain.

You built the brain you have today and will continue to refine and remodel it with every action, thought, and feeling and every interaction with the people, the experiences, and the environment around you.

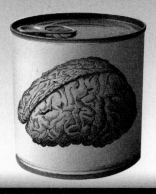

CHAPTER THREE

Your Brain Growing Older
What to Expect in a Healthy Aging Brain

There is quite a bit of good news about your brain as it ages, Now, it's not as good as some anti-aging enthusiasts proclaim. The fact is that there is no way stop to aging or reverse its effects.

Just like the rest of your body, your brain is growing old. And in the same way, how well it ages varies from person to person. It's affected by your genes, life experiences and lifestyle, and exposure to toxins, illnesses, and accidents. Some changes, like wrinkles, are unavoidable.

Your body and brain will slowly fade, but before they do, there is plenty to rejoice in. We used to think that progressive mental decline was inevitable, but that's not so. For openers, researchers are finding that in most healthy people, our cognitive abilities do not drop dramatically with age; the effects are subtle, and our ability to make good decisions may increase (albeit it may take us a bit longer to get there).

Yes, we do experience some memory loss as the years pass, especially minor forgetfulness and difficulty retrieving words while speaking (and finding those darn keys). Our ability to quickly manipulate numbers, objects, and images may also decline some in our later years. But even at age 80, general intelligence and verbal abilities are not much worse than they were decades earlier, unless there is some serious illness affecting the brain.

The average brain can absorb quite a bit before it begins to falter, and most brains go on functioning pretty well to just before the end. Even the brains of many of those who reach and pass the age of 100 years appear to retain abilities: they can communicate and converse and enjoy life.

Other brains do fall prey to bad luck—to accidents, injuries, disease, or genetics. (See Chapter Four, "What Can Go Wrong.") But researchers have found that even with severe brain changes, you may be functioning fine: autopsies have found the brains of some people who appeared healthy and happy into old age actually showed signs of damage, loss, and disease associated with Alzheimer's. Healthy aging is possible for many, if not most, of us. If you are lucky in your genetics and life experiences and you take care of some simple health measures (even starting now), your brain will last as long as you will. (See the chapters in Part Three, "How to Optimize Your Aging Brain.")

Your mature older brain is more plastic than we used to think, proving wrong that outdated dictum, "Old dogs can't learn new tricks." The older brain generally learns new pursuits more slowly than its younger self (and can't reach the peaks of expertise in a given field as if it had started in its youth), but you can maintain your cognitive performance through effort, forestalling some of the declines in cognition that come with advancing age.

The Usual Effects of Aging

Not surprisingly, the changes in your brain are very much the same as those seen in the rest of your aging body. It does slow down, just like an aging athlete. But just like that older athlete, you may not need all that top performance power of the past.

Here's what the average healthy brain can expect as it ages:

- Sometime around 40 or 50, your brain will begin to show subtle signs of aging that can be seen on a brain scan, but you may not notice any change in function.
- As it ages, your brain becomes lighter and smaller, losing volume, some neurons, and some white matter. The normal brains of elders are up to 15 percent smaller than younger brains.
- Your neuronal networks will begin to run more slowly in later years due in part to a decrease of the myelin, or white matter, that helps zip information among your neurons.
- Your brain becomes less nimble. Multitasking—switching back and forth between (or among!) tasks—is not as easy for older brains. And that may not be such a bad thing: several studies show that any brain at any age may not be happy rapidly switching focus.
- The elder brain functions differently from younger ones. For the easy tasks, older brain activity is very similar to its younger self, but tougher challenges call on more brain areas than previously. Seniors activate several frontal brain regions that the younger brain did not.
- Old injuries take a toll. Not much to be done about that: just like overstressed joints, brains that have been injured in the past by accidents and illness may function less well as they age, but often we can compensate.
- There's increased risk for nonbrain illnesses that can impair function. Dementia may be a by-product of other conditions connected

with aging, such as heart disease, diabetes, Parkinson's disease, and stroke.

- Your brain needs to be worked, especially as it ages, to stay at its personal best. Persistent and continued exercise—physical, social, and mental—spurs brain growth and is associated with a perkier brain and a decreased risk of dementia.

- The potential for happiness increases. The possessors of older brains report that they are happier in their 70s than at any other time since their early 20s, and they have more positive than negative memories.

- Sexual desire still sets flames in the neuronal networks pretty much regardless of age.

Do the Brains of Men and Women Age Differently?

It's hard to say which gender has the better-preserved brain. Women live longer than men and seem to do better healthwise from the get-go. But does that apply to brain as well as body?

The death rates for women are lower than those for men at all ages—even before birth. About 115 males are conceived for every 100 females, but their numbers start declining immediately due to stillbirths and miscarriages: about 104 boys are born alive for every 100 girls, and more boys than girls die in infancy. (This is not true in cultures that favor males and suppress the birth of girl babies by abortion or by infanticide.) Every year after that, more males die, so that by age 25 or so, women are in the majority. Women also outlive men by about two years on the average.

Therefore, it stands to reason that more women end up with dementia and Alzheimer's disease. Two-thirds of those with the disease, 3.4 million, are women, even though they are not at a greater risk of developing it. But perhaps if men lived longer, that would not be so: more would succumb to Alzheimer's. A recent study finds that mild cognitive impairment—problems with memory or thinking that is often a precursor of Alzheimer's disease—is 1.5 times higher in men compared to women.

A 2010 Mayo Clinic study of aging interviewed 2,050 people between the ages of 70 to 89 in Olmstead County, Minnesota, about their medical history and tested them on their memory and thinking skills. About 76 percent of those tested had normal memory and thinking skills, nearly 14 percent of all participants had mild cognitive impairment, and about 10 percent had dementia. Nineteen percent of men had mild cognitive impairment compared to 14 percent of women. People in the study who had a low level of education or were never married also had a higher rate of mild cognitive impairment.

The researchers speculate that factors related to gender play a role in brain health. Estrogen, the female hormone, could be protective. Or it could be that men have cognitive decline earlier in life, but more gradually, whereas women may transition from normal memory directly to dementia at a later age but more quickly.

Indeed, there is a difference between the sexes in disease patterns, with women having more chronic nonfatal conditions, such as arthritis, osteoporosis, and autoimmune disorders, and men having more fatal conditions, such as heart disease and cancer. It could be that women live with their diseases, while men die from them.

How Memory Works: The Short Version

Memory loss is the big bugaboo of aging and for most of us, the canary in the coal mine: an early warning system that something is about to go terribly wrong in the brain.

A brief primer on how memory works, and why forgetting is important, might allay some of those fears.

Memory is essential for our very identity: we need it to create our sense of self, and some think immortality is the memory of you

THE AMAZING HEALING BRAIN

Even with enormous injuries and insults, your brain may be able to repair or adjust itself to allow healthy sections to take up the slack:

- You can live with half a brain. People who have had part of their brain removed to stop severe and debilitating epilepsy seizures manage surprisingly well, especially children. In Parkinson's disease, some areas of the brain involving motor control are surgically destroyed, which can help relieve symptoms.
- Your brain can recover from major, even devastating, injury. Journalist Bob Woodruff, seriously brain-injured covering combat in Iraq at age 45, made a near-miraculous recovery after extensive therapy—and returned to work.
- Your brain can recover from stroke, depending on how severe the damage, the part of the brain affected, and how quickly you get treatment. After extensive therapy, it may rewire itself and recover many functions.
- Exercise—physical, mental, and social—helps repair and maintain your brain. It lowers stress, which damages the brain; encourages neurons to grow and make more connections; and spurs the growth of new brain cells in some areas and provokes more white matter.
- Deep brain stimulation imparted through electrodes implanted in the brain has helped many brains ailing from depression, Parkinson's disease, and epilepsy and shows promise of stimulating other brain repairs.

that is held by others. It may seem that memory is all about the past, but in fact, memory is about the present and the future, helping us move through the now. It's the process of acquiring and storing information from our experiences that we will need to navigate similar situations in the future. Our very survival may depend on it. No wonder losing memory is one of the tragedies of Alzheimer's and other diseases of dementia.

It's tempting to think of memories as bits of specific information stored in a specific place that you can just retrieve at will. However, your memories are not held neatly inside individual neurons. Instead, they are created when messages are sent across synapses, the tiny gaps between neurons, from the outgoing axon on one neuron to the dendrite on another neuron that receives information. A memory is held in the connections this network makes and is firmly established when a network of synapses is strengthened—temporarily for a short-term memory and more-or-less permanently for a long-term one. Over time, this net of memories can be strengthened further, weakened, or broken, depending on a combination of your brain chemistry, your genes, your actions, and whether you acquire a brain-damaging disease or injury.

There are many different kinds of memory, stored in different ways and housed in different places in the brain. Short-term memory, a form of working memory, is fleeting—say, when you are surfing the Net and need to recall what you've just seen for thirty seconds or less. Then the memory is discarded or transferred to long-term memory. The transition is called consolidation. The hippocampus, among other structures in the medial temporal lobe, is key to converting short- to long-term memories, and it's an area that is damaged in Alzheimer's disease.

Long-term memories are complex and can be both conscious and unconscious. Explicit memory, or declarative memory, is what most of us think about as memory. It requires conscious thought to recall, say, the name of your first lover or textbook knowledge (such as the parts of the brain that process memories). It's primarily explicit memory that fails in Alzheimer's and most other kinds of dementia.

Implicit, or nondeclarative, memory includes rote memory involving habits and motor skills. It doesn't require conscious thought for most of us to recall how to brush our teeth or how to ride a bicycle. Those with advanced Alzheimer's who no longer recognize their children may still play the piano beautifully. Scientists have long puzzled over why and how we choose to retain some information and not others. Your brain is constantly filtering incoming messages, deciding what information to keep, and how to go about it. Sometimes it takes repetition—for example, to learn that $6 \times 7 = 42$, to memorize the periodic table of elements, or to learn your social security number and the passwords to your social network and bank accounts.

And sometimes, says memory researcher R. Douglas Fields, we don't need to be told twice. A single potent experience can burn an experience indelibly into your brain, and that's never more true than when the memory is connected with survival. Fields, chief of the Nervous System Development and Plasticity Section at the National Institute of Child Health and Human Development, has been studying memory making for years and writing about it for *Scientific American.* He gives this example of a childhood memory that persists. There's a shortcut to school that crosses the old Dugan place, overgrown with weeds and littered with junk cars. Just as you set foot on the property, Old Man Dugan throws open his screen door and two pit bulls charge you, snarling with teeth bared. You run for your life, narrowly escaping. The next morning and forever after, you take the long route instead. Returning years later to that place, your heart still races, even though Dugan and the dogs are long gone. And in the years since the incident, you have developed a lifelong phobia for dogs.

Why? Because, Fields says, from a biological or evolutionary perspective, memory is about the future: it keeps only what you need. There's no survival value in having a recording system in your brain that accurately retains each and every event and experience. (Anyone struggling to manage burgeoning e-mail files knows the solution is not a bigger inbox; it's to delete the files that aren't needed.)

The trick for your brain is to weigh the minute-to-minute experiences and instantly pick out the ones to keep for reference and the ones to discard. Now the survival value of certain events is immediately apparent, and memories of them are socked away permanently. After the Dugan episode, Fields says, you'll always recognize the danger in the presence of an onrushing dog.

Why then do we have trouble making new memories or retaining short-term ones when we are older? It has a lot to do, Fields says, with the gradual loss of myelin, or white matter.

Why White Matter Matters

As your brain grows older, it shrinks somewhat, losing gray matter (neurons) and white matter (myelin). The loss of white matter seems to matter more because it plays the key role in connectivity, and our ability to think depends on our brain circuitry.

The loss of white matter, which allows electrical signals to travel through the brain quickly and efficiently, means it takes longer to connect a face with a name, a book with an author, or any other facts. Its loss also makes the brain "noisier," that is, less able to sort out important from unimportant input.

But myelin loss, according to new research, should come with an asterisk: most of it seems to occur in specific parts of the brain—the parts responsible for learning new things. The part responsible for long-term memory shows no such loss, as most of us can testify.

As researchers learn more about myelin, they have discovered that some specific protein molecules may stop axons from sprouting and forming new connections that send out information. Martin E. Schwab, a brain researcher at the University of Zurich, found several myelin proteins that cause young sprouts from axons to wither instantly on contact. And the startling good news is that when this protein, called Nogo-A, is neutralized, animals with a spinal cord injury can repair their damaged connections and recover sensation and movement. Then Stephen M. Strittmatter of Yale found that wiring and rewiring the brains of animals through experience could be helped by blocking signals from Nogo-A: when these were disrupted in old mice, the critters rewired connections.

This is still being studied and could have a major impact on aging, as well as recovery from devastating injuries, as myelination is largely finished in a person's 20s and begins to degrade after our 50s.

The Aging Brain: Is It Less Connected?

The connectivity spurred by white matter is also crucial to how your different brain regions are able to communicate with each other, called cross-talk. As it dwindles, so does that function.

In one study, scientists used functional magnetic resonance imaging (fMRI) to monitor activity in the fronts and backs of brains while study participants performed several cognitive and memory exercises, such as determining whether certain words referred to living or nonliving objects. As they answered, researchers were able to see which brain parts were operating in sync. In older brains, communication between brain regions appeared to have dramatically declined.

They fingered the potential reason for the dip by doing further brain scans using diffusion tensor imaging, a technique that gauges how well white matter is functioning by monitoring water movement along the axonal bundles. If communication is strong, water flows as if cascading down a celery stalk, says Randy Buckner, a cognitive neuroscientist at Harvard; if it is disrupted, the pattern looks more like a drop of dye in a water bucket that has scattered in all directions. The latter was more evident in the older group, an indication that their white matter had lost some of its integrity.

The older crowd's performance on memory and cognitive skill tests correlated with white matter loss: the seniors who did poorly compared to their younger peers had more white matter loss. Researchers speculate that age-related depletion of neurotransmitters (the chemical signals sent between neurons), as well as the shrinking of gray matter, contributes to dimming memory and cognitive skills.

Now that doesn't contradict findings that the brain remains plastic throughout middle and old age—if your brain remains active. For example, studies show that mental and physical exercise into a person's 60s, 70s, 80s, and beyond seems to delay the onset of Alzheimer's disease. (See the chapters in Part Three, "How to Optimize Your Aging Brain.")

Older brains can continue to learn, but they are engaged in a different kind of learning. Intensive training causes neurons to fire—to generate an electrical charge and release neurotransmitters—and that activity has been shown to stimulate myelination, which appears to be connected to better cognition. Perhaps someday, when we fully understand when and why white matter forms, we can devise treatments to harness it and preserve it as it—and we—grow old.

Forgetting May Be Vital to Remembering

Forgetting is not all bad, and in fact it may be a useful skill. The next time a word or name stays frustratingly out of reach, consider this: your brain may be just doing its job. Forgetting not only helps the brain conserve energy; it also improves short-term memory and recall of important details, according to two Stanford University studies.

Scientists had students study 240 word pairs and then instructed them to memorize only a small subset of the list, asking them to selectively retain some pairs and mentally discard others. Then the researchers performed magnetic resonance imaging (MRI) scans while testing them to see how well they had learned all the pairs. Those who were best at summing up the retained pairs were also the worst at remembering the ones to discard, suggesting that they were better at unconsciously filtering out unwanted memories—and their MRI scans showed reduced activity in the prefrontal cortex, an area associated with detecting and resolving memory conflicts. "When we want to remember things that are relevant, we put in much less neural effort if we have forgotten the things that are irrelevant," says psychologist Anthony Wagner, a coauthor of the study.

The findings suggest that suppressing memory helps us conserve energy and improve efficiency, which goes along with research showing that efficient brains think faster. A second study reveals that working memory (that short-term memory) benefits from an inhibition of long-term memory. Working memory is a kind of temporary depository for handing incoming information, while long-term memory is, as the name says, more lasting.

Working with mice, researchers used X-rays or genetic techniques to stop the formation of new neurons in the hippocampus, an area important for consolidating long-term memories. These mice were better at maze-related working memory tasks than normal mice, suggesting to researchers that impairing one form of memory improves another form, says Gaël Malleret, a neuroscientist at Columbia University and coauthor of the study.

So if you accidentally called your neighbor by the wrong name, don't worry: your brain probably just chose to dump his name in favor of a more crucial fact, such as where you left those darn keys.

Five Things Most People Get Wrong About Memory

While you worry about the slips and gaps in your aging memory, here's some consolation: human memory has been shown again and again to be far from perfect at any age. We overlook big things, forget details, and conflate events. One famous experiment even demonstrated that many people asked to watch a video of a basketball game failed to notice or remember when a person wearing a gorilla suit walked right through the middle of the scene.

A 2011 nationwide survey of fifteen hundred U.S. adults shows that many people continue to have the wrong idea about how we remember and what we forget. So why does a temporary gap in remembering after midlife cause such consternation? It's because we seem to have some inaccurate ideas about memory: it never was as good as most of us seem to think it was.

Here are five common incorrect assumptions about memory that experts say should be forgotten:

1. *Myth: Memory works like a video camera, recording the world around us onto a mental tape that we can later replay.* Nearly two-thirds (63 percent) of those in the random telephone survey said that they agreed with this model of a passively recorded memory. This notion runs counter to research that has shown events to be recalled based on goals and expectations, and findings that memory retrieval is a constructive process that can be shaped by assumptions and beliefs, noted study authors Daniel Simons, of the University of Illinois, and Christopher Chabris, of Union College, both of them psychology professors.

2. *Myth: An unexpected occurrence is likely to be noticed, even when people's attention is elsewhere.* More than three-quarters (77.5 percent) of people thought that this would be the case. Clearly they are unfamiliar with the gorilla suit study. That work and other research have shown that unexpected—and even preposterous—details frequently go unnoticed and thus do not make it into memory. Aside from a false certainty that one would notice someone wearing an oversized primate costume, this presumption could have some serious implications for the legal system and eyewitness testimony.

3. *Myth: Hypnosis can improve memory, especially when assisting a witness in recalling details associated with a crime.* Most memory experts disagree with this statement, but more than half (55.4 percent) of the surveyed public thought that it was accurate. Courts

have already steered away from accepting testimony gathered through hypnosis. And many studies have demonstrated that people under hypnosis—and even those who are not—can often be led by questioners to "recall" things that never occurred.

4. *Myth: Amnesia sufferers usually cannot remember their identity or name.* Although soap operas might lead you to conclude otherwise, most common forms of amnesia interfere with the formation of new long-term memories, usually as a result of a major brain injury. The researchers cite the movie *Memento* (2000) as a reasonably accurate portrayal of the condition; it shows a man unable to store new memories and able to remember an event for only a few minutes. But most popular portraits "depict amnesia as something more like a much rarer fugue state in which someone cannot remember who they are and suddenly take leave of their home and work," they noted. Perhaps because of the prevalence of this blank-stare amnesia in television and movies, a whopping 82.7 percent of those surveyed shared this (incorrect) view of the condition.

5. *Myth: Memories are forever.* The survey found that nearly half (47.6 percent) of respondents said that once a memory is formed, it is set in stone. This is also not true, say the researchers: "Our memories can change even if we don't realize they have changed," Simons said. That's why it's called re-membering. Along these lines, more than a third (37.1 percent) of people thought that "confident" testimony from a witness should be adequate for a criminal conviction. Yet defendants who were later shown to be innocent as a result of DNA testing had originally been convicted based on a faulty identification by an eyewitness.

If there's one thing to remember about these findings, it's that "people tend to place greater faith in the accuracy, completeness and vividness of their memories than they probably should," Simons said.

To see how you and other readers measure up to the experts, the authors of the study, Christopher Chabris and Daniel Simons (who also wrote the book *The Invisible Gorilla*), have created an online quiz that also shows the rates of correct—and incorrect—responses to the survey question (to see it, go to http://www.theinvisiblegorilla.com/).

The Good News: Slower Is Sometimes Better

So your aging brain is slowing down—but that might not be so bad. In fact, in some cases, it could be a downright advantage. Several studies suggest that an aging brain might be more accurate, more thoughtful, more social, and better able to use more of its parts.

As your brain ages, perception of sights, sounds, and smells take a bit longer, and laying down new information into memory becomes more difficult. The ability to retrieve memories quickly also slides, and it is sometimes harder to concentrate and maintain attention.

But, studies show, although perception and reaction time do indeed take longer, that slowing down doesn't necessarily undermine mental acuity. Indeed, evidence shows that older brains can be as mentally fit as younger ones: they just work in different and creative ways to compensate for some kinds of declines in ways that can keep seniors nearly as sharp as youngsters, especially when tackling challenging tasks.

A significant advantage of an older brain is being able to tap into its extensive store of knowledge and experience. Perhaps the biggest trick is to use both hemispheres simultaneously to handle tasks for which younger brains rely predominantly on only one side.

Cindy Lustig of the University of Michigan, Ann Arbor, used fMRI imaging to observe the brains of young adults (aged 18 to 30) and seniors (aged 65 to 92) as they tackled simple and difficult mental exercises. For the easy tasks, brain activity was very similar, but tougher challenges prompted differences. The seniors activated several frontal brain regions that the younger brains did not. In addition, the younger people "turned off" parts of the brain during the tasks, whereas the elders kept those regions active. Using both sides of the brain gives elders a tactical edge, even if the pure speed of each hemisphere's processing is slower.

In an animal study, Michela Gallagher of Johns Hopkins compared the brains of 6-month-old rats with 2-year-old rats, who are elderly by rat standards. Her team also divided the elder rats into age-impaired and age-unimpaired groups. When Gallagher compared the synapses among the aged rats, she found that the impaired rats had lost the ability to adjust the activity of synapses appropriately but that the unimpaired rats had not. These connections are how memories are formed and preserved, and the study suggests that healthy older brains can function quite well.

USE THOSE WORDS, OR LOSE THEM

We all know the maddening experience of not being able to think of a certain word that is undoubtedly in our repertoire—and our memory—if only we could retrieve it.

Researchers have discovered an association between a specific region in the neural language system and these tip-of-the-tongue (TOT) experiences that are a normal part of aging. Deborah Burke of Pomona College and her team found that TOT moments became more frequent as gray matter density in the left insula declined. This is an area of the brain implicated in sound processing and production.

The findings support a proposal by Burke and her colleagues predicting that when we do not use a word often, the connections among all its various representations in the brain become weak. "Words aren't stored as a unit," she says. "Instead you have the sound information connected to semantic information, connected to grammatical information, and so on. But the sounds are much more vulnerable to decay over time than other kinds of information, and that leads to the TOT experience." Good news for some of us who spend much time alone and talk to ourselves: it has a purpose.

Older brains also may think more. A study at the University of Dortmund in Germany found that elders presented with new computer exercises paused longer before reacting and took longer to complete the tasks. Yet they made 50 percent fewer errors, probably because of their more deliberate pace.

Look at it this way: Think of a test to determine who can type a paragraph "better"—a 16 year old who glides along at sixty words per minute but then has to double-back to correct a number of mistakes, or a 70 year old who strikes keys at only forty words per minute but spends less time fixing errors. In the end, if "better" is defined as completing a clean paragraph, both people may end up taking the same amount of time.

Computerized tests also show that accuracy can offset speed. In one so-called distraction exercise, people were told to look at a screen, wait for an arrow that pointed in a certain direction to appear, and then use a mouse to click on it as soon as it appeared on the screen. Just before the correct symbol appeared, however, the computer displayed numerous other arrows aimed in various other directions. Although younger subjects cut through the confusion faster when the properly positioned arrow suddenly popped up, in their haste they more frequently clicked on an incorrect symbol. When tests such as language comprehension and processing don't depend on speed, older test takers are equally capable. In these cases, the elders used the brain's available resources in a different way. Neurologists at the Cognitive Neurology and Alzheimer's Disease Center at Northwestern University came to this conclusion after analyzing fifty test subjects ranging in age from 23 to 78. The subjects lay down in an MRI machine and were asked to concentrate on two different lists of printed words posted side by side in front of them. By looking at the lists, they were to find pairs of words that were similar in meaning or spelling.

The eldest participants did just as well on the tests as the youngest ones. And yet the MRI scans showed that the elders' left frontal and temporal lobes and certain visual centers, which together are responsible for language recognition and interpretation, were much less active. The researchers did find that the older people had more activity in brain regions responsible for attentiveness, such as the posterior cingulate cortex. Darren Gitelman, who headed the study, concluded that older brains solved the problems just as effectively as younger ones but by different means.

Similar adaptation seems to aid memory. In 2003 Mara Mather and her colleagues at the University of California, Santa Cruz, found that older adults who performed well on memory tests used a process of comparing bits of memories that was different from the memory-recollection mechanisms that younger people used.

It appears that slower processing speed, and not memory lapses, could account for communication problems in older brains, especially when the older brain is engaged in two or more tasks at the same time. In the five-year Language Across the Life Span Project funded by the National Institute on Aging, researchers led by Susan Kemper have identified the aging brain's slower processing speed as the prime candidate in typical communication problems of healthy older adults.

But she and her colleagues also discovered that older folks appear to think more. When young and older adults were asked to keep a cursor on a moving target and answer questions, the younger participants did do better staying on target. But Kemper noticed another pattern: the younger group tended to focus on keeping up with the target and thus gave briefer answers, whereas the older adults focused on giving more complex and thoughtful answers.

The bottom line: neuronal networks remain surprisingly flexible, or plastic. Animal experiments prove that an intact nerve cell can take over the function of a neighboring nerve cell that has become damaged or has withered with time. The brain creates ways to keep itself sharp by making these kinds of adjustments on a widespread scale over time.

Eventually your brain may lose some of that plasticity. Researchers are discovering more about why an aging brain eventually becomes less resilient and able to store new experiences, and they are exploring ways to help older brains stay sharp and perhaps even recover from some decline. Research has shown that physical and mental activity, along with some basic health and lifestyle actions, help to keep brains supple and are associated with a lower risk of developing dementia.

More Easily Distracted: Why Multitasking Is a Task

You know that glitch you get when you leave the living room and head off for the kitchen and forget what you wanted when you get there? It may not be due completely to memory issues but rather to an interaction between memory and attention. The older brain may slow down because it's more easily distracted, and processing speeds slacken along with the ability to block out irrelevant information.

In one study, Adam Gazzaley of the University of California, San Francisco, and his colleagues asked two groups—one made up of 19 to 33 year olds and the other of 60 to 72 year olds—to perform a memory task. The researchers used electroencephalography to record electrical signals from the participants' brains in milliseconds during the task.

During the first 200 milliseconds after exposure, the older group could not screen out distracting stimuli as well as the younger adults could. The ability to ignore wasn't abolished; it was just delayed. By then, however, the irrelevant information had interfered with the memory task, making the older group less accurate overall than the younger group. But not all older adults are more distracted compared to younger adults, Gazzaley notes. When he divided the older group in half according to performance scores, only the low scorers had the problem.

While we can hit a glitch in multitasking at any age, Gazzaley and colleagues have a theory about why multitasking gets difficult with passing years. It seems our older brains can't switch back and forth as easily between what they call working memory and maintenance memory. Working memory is when you hold information in your mind for a usually brief period, such as that walk from the living room to the kitchen or while transferring a phone number from your address book to your smart phone. It's also needed to follow a conversation and, heaven forbid, remember what you just said while giving a speech or discourse. Maintenance memory, or long-term memory, is what you store away for later.

In a recent study using fMRI, the researchers had two age groups view a scene for about fourteen seconds, then interrupted them with an image of a face and some questions, and then asked them to recall the original scene. The older group (median age 69.1) had more trouble recalling the original scene than the younger group (median age 24.5).

When they examined the fMRIs, researchers saw why: when interrupted, the brains of both groups disengaged from a memory maintenance network and reallocated brain resources toward processing the interruption. However, after the interruption, the younger adults were able to easily reconnect with the memory maintenance network, while the older adults failed both to ignore the interruption and reestablish the neural network associated with the disrupted memory.

They say the ability to ignore distractions is key to memory formation, and becomes more difficult with age—and with the increasingly complex and distracting world we live in.

Incidentally, other scientists have noted that our basic brain structure could explain why people have difficulty multitasking at any age. When we do two things at the same time, our brain divides the work in half, literally: each hemisphere concentrates on one task, reports a 2010 study in *Science*. Researchers measuring brain activity in volunteers who were performing letter-pairing tests found that when subjects had to deal with two streams of letters—concurrently performing two pairing tasks—the activity in one half of the brain corresponded to one task, and the activity in the other half corresponded to the other.

The study might explain why people are notoriously poor at doing three or more things simultaneously. After two tasks, we run out of hemispheres. So that may be part of the point, which is . . . Wait, don't tell me. Oh yes, multitasking.

PART TWO

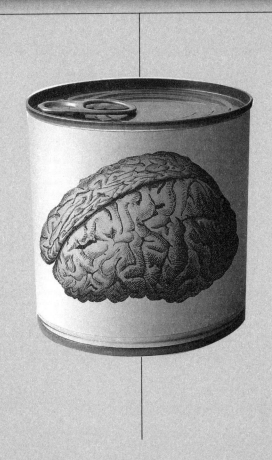

Threats to Your Brain

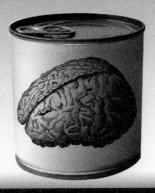

CHAPTER FOUR

What Can Go Wrong

Your brain is one of your most resilient organs—and perhaps the only one that still has its original parts: most of your brain cells are as old as you are.

With some exceptions, your brain functions pretty well and lasts as long as you do. In fact, your cognitive abilities may outlast your knees, hips, vision, and hearing. In short, your brain is in this for the long haul. And don't forget your brain's amazing ability to repair itself, bypassing damaged areas and even growing new neurons (neurogenesis) in some areas.

As we well know, a gradual decline in some mental functions is a normal part of aging. Just as your body slows and ages, so does your brain. But there are accidents, diseases, and conditions that can incapacitate you and your brain at any time. And although dementia, depression, and other brain disorders are not part of normal aging, the risk of these increases with age.

Aging, alas, is one risk factor you just can't dodge, and sometimes aging is more than just years passing. It's the accumulation of diseases and disasters over time: illnesses and past infections, old head injuries from falls, accidents, and sports. Genetics also plays a role, though in most cases much less than you may think: it's complex and dependent on many factors, so even if dementia, Parkinson's disease, or other ailments of aging run in your family, you may not develop these.

There are many unknowns. It's important to remember that just like other disorders, brain disease can strike without apparent reason.

THREATS TO YOUR AGING BRAIN

Here's a summary of the most common things that could go wrong or contribute to problems with your brain as it ages (more detailed sections on each follows). In some cases, treatment may be able to slow or stop the progression of symptoms.

- *Alzheimer's disease and other dementias.* There are several types and causes of dementia, the decline of memory and thinking due to damage to brain cells and neural networks. Alzheimer's disease is by far the most prevalent, accounting for up to 80 percent of dementias.

- *Mild cognitive impairment (MCI)* is characterized by memory and thinking problems greater than those associated with normal aging, but it is not as severe as dementia and in some cases may be slowed or halted. It affects up to an estimated 42 percent of those over the age of 65.

- *Stroke* does its damage by interrupting blood flow and starving the brain of oxygen and glucose. Risk increases at age 55 and more than doubles each decade after that, with three-quarters of all strokes occurring after age 65.

- *Parkinson's disease,* a gradual loss of motor control, affects about 4 million people worldwide, or 1 percent of the population older than 60, the average age of onset.

You can live a life rife with unhealthy activities and practices known to contribute to poor brain health and die with your mental faculties intact. Or you can do everything right and end up with a brain-disabling condition.

Even with the best of intentions and the best-lived life, factors beyond your control can increase your risk of cognitive impairment and dementia.

Life isn't always fair or even reasonable, and there is no point in blaming or applauding yourself (or your genes) for the state of your brain today.

- *Diabetes,* an inability to produce or process insulin, affects 25.8 million people in the United States—10.9 million, or 26.9 percent, of all people over age 65—and it may nearly double your risk of developing Alzheimer's disease.

- *Traumatic brain injury (TBI)* more than doubles the risk of dementia, and falls are a leading cause of TBI and an increased risk as we age. Brain injury leading to cognitive problems also comes from vehicular accidents and sports injuries and military combat.

- *Depression* is not a part of normal aging in healthy elders and can be treated. It can also be a sign that something else is wrong, such as an infection, dementia, brain tumor, Parkinson's disease, and other conditions, some of them treatable or reversible.

- *Past injuries and illnesses,* such as cancer and its treatments (chemotherapy and radiation) or past head injuries, may affect cognition, and the effects may increase with age and can mimic or contribute to dementia and mental fuzziness. Some chronic illnesses, such as multiple sclerosis and lupus, also contribute to mental fuzziness.

- *Medication effects or interactions* can contribute to or mimic dementia and may be overlooked. Indeed, some may be prescribed by your doctors in good faith, so medication should be regularly checked.

When Your Brain Needs Help: How Can You Tell?

Forgot your reading glasses—again? Can't find your keys—and you left the tea kettle on the stove and burned out the bottom? Again. And what was it you just went into the bedroom to get?

We find ways to cope: multiple pairs of reading glasses, a second set of keys hung on a hook right by the door (with a spare at the neighbor's), and an electric kettle with an automatic shut-off.

But enough of these episodes can make a person begin to wonder: *Am I losing my memory and my mind?*

The fact is, as most of us know all too well, such minor forgetfulness can happen at any age. Remember when you left your lunch on the school bus in third grade and your mittens at the playground? Back then and well into midlife, such minor lapses are unlikely to cause you to jump to the conclusion that you have a serious brain problem.

But past midlife, such events become more sinister. Forgetting a name or date, losing your way in a strange city, missing an appointment—we worry. The specter of dementia haunts us all as we live longer and see our parents, our friends, and even our former presidents and sports heroes succumb to dementia.

So when you find yourself forgetting things, then—*Omigosh, it must be the onset of Alzheimer's disease!* Men and women who are middle aged or older are quick to diagnose themselves with inevitable dementia. But there is no need to panic if lately you have forgotten an appointment or a friend's birthday. The reasons for memory lapses are usually much less dire than suspected. Almost any form of stress or emotional pressure can cause memory problems, a well-documented fact that many people never consider, as can a number of seemingly unrelated physical conditions such as an infection or even dehydration. Figuring out the source of mild cognitive symptoms and relieving them can work wonders.

So how can you distinguish what's normal aging from when a brain needs help? A certain amount of change and slower functioning is to be expected. But what foreshadows dementia? When does TOT, that tip-of-the-tongue memory lapse, become short-term memory loss?

Even the geriatricians who specialize in caring for the health needs of the elderly have a hard time marking the point at which some diminishing of skills and function becomes a disease. But it's an important issue. Even though there are no cures and few truly effective treatments for Alzheimer's disease so far, diagnosing the precursors of dementia as early as possible is important because some kinds of dementia can be helped, such as those associated with heart disease and other coexisting conditions. Also, these symptoms may not be dementia at all, but the result of other conditions with similar symptoms, such as depression or medication errors that can be treated and even reversed. Mental changes don't always mean dementia. (See "Maybe It's Not Alzheimer's Disease" later in this chapter.)

Your own expectations may be to blame for "bad" memory, when any number of neurological and psychiatric conditions could be causing problems. Emotional issues can make a person more forgetful. Adapting to the inevitable losses of aging—the death of mate and friends—leaves some people feeling temporarily confused or forgetful.

Tremendous media attention has been focused on memory loss and Alzheimer's disease, so that some of us, including our doctors, might be a bit overly sensitized and find symptoms everywhere. But just because you can't recall the answer to a question on *Jeopardy* or the Sunday crossword puzzle doesn't mean you're on the way to incipient dementia; at most, it may mean that you need to brush up on your trivia. In the end, physical and mental exercise, a healthy diet, proper rest, and stress reduction are the best ways to keep your memory sharp as you grow older.

If you are concerned about what appears to be inexplicable memory deterioration, then you might go to a neurologist, a geriatrician, or a clinic specializing in memory issues for an evaluation.

SIGNS OF MENTAL DECLINE

It's true that early diagnosis of mental fuzziness is important because mild cognitive impairment (MCI) or symptoms that look like dementia may not be so and could be treated and even reversed. Here are some of signs of memory loss and confusion that suggest you may need to seek professional help:

- Asking the same questions repeatedly
- Repeating the same story word for word multiple times
- Forgetting how to do basic tasks that you once performed easily such as cooking, making repairs, and playing cards
- Problems paying bills or balancing a checkbook (if these weren't difficult before)
- Getting lost in familiar places
- Neglecting personal hygiene, such as bathing or dressing in clean clothes while insisting on having taken a bath or put on a new outfit
- Relying on someone else to make decisions, such as what to buy at a supermarket or where to go next, that were easily handled in the past
- Frequent falls or difficulty with balance

None of these alone or even in combination is a sure sign of decline. After all, we all have a bad day now and then when we can't think straight. But anyone who shows several of these should see a specialist for an examination.

Specialists will take detailed information and interview you to determine whether you actually have a memory problem—and if so, why. They'll examine your health history and your past and current medications. A neurologist will test your reflexes and reactions for any physical problems. Psychological tests will assess whether you can draw conclusions adeptly, handle numbers correctly, and name objects. Temporal and spatial orientation tasks will test your abstract thinking, judgment, and verbal and mathematical abilities, as well as your ability to draw geometrical figures. All these can help identify memory problems—or put to rest your concerns about them.

Looking at your general health, a geriatric specialist can determine whether aging or some other factor may be the root of some problems. Researchers are discovering seemingly minor changes in your life might bring about significant memory improvement.

The Darkness of Dementia

Dementia used to be thought a normal part of aging. That's a mistaken belief, but it may prevent patients, their families, and even their doctors from checking into the many conditions or situations that can contribute to what looks like Alzheimer's disease.

It's true that dementias are the most common, and perhaps most dreaded, age-related brain issue. There are several types, with Alzheimer's disease by far the most prevalent: it accounts for up to 80 percent of dementias, and it's estimated nearly half of those over age 85 will develop it. (For a detailed discussion of dementia, see Chapter Five, "Alzheimer's Disease.")

There is, for now, no effective treatment for Alzheimer's disease and no definitive cause. However, lifestyle issues are increasingly being associated with this and other cognitive issues. (See Part Three, "How to Optimize Your Aging Brain.") In addition, billions are being spent on extensive research.

Most kinds of dementia are marked by abnormalities or damage that can be seen in the ailing brain. Vascular dementia, the second most common type, develops when blood flow is impaired to parts of the brain and brain cells die. It's typically caused by a stroke or a series of strokes or other changes in the brain's blood supply. Quick treatment may minimize some brain damage (see "Stroke: The Brain Attack" later in this chapter). Dementia with Lewy bodies, characterized by abnormal protein deposits, progresses much like Alzheimer's disease.

Frontotemporal dementia affects the front and side brain especially and is characterized by language difficulty and changes in personality. Dementia may also come about after a long bout with a serious chronic illness: those with Parkinson's disease may develop dementia in the later stages of the disease, for example. Inflammation kills brain cells. Repeated brain injuries (such as from blows to the head), alcoholism, and AIDS also damage brain tissue and may lead to dementia.

MAYBE IT'S NOT ALZHEIMER'S DISEASE

Dementia may be the first fear when things begin to go wrong mentally, but before deciding it must be a brain disease, experts suggest considering some of these conditions that mimic dementia—and may be treatable and reversible:

- *Overmedication and drug interactions.* Many elders are taking a dozen or so medications daily for a variety of conditions, and all of them have side effects. One of the best-selling drug classes, statins, has been known to cause dementia-like symptoms in rare cases in some people.
- *Dehydration,* which can cause headache, confusion, and memory issues.
- *High fever and untreated infections.* Low-level infections may go undiagnosed and cause confusion.
- *Vitamin and nutritional deficiencies,* especially of the B and D vitamins.
- *Heart disease,* especially high blood pressure, and vascular diseases can cause confusion.
- *Untreated chronic conditions* such as thyroid imbalances, diabetes, or a brain tumor.
- *Alcoholism, or just too much to drink.* Age makes us more susceptible to the effects of alcohol, which also contributes to depression.
- *Depression, stress, and anxiety.* These are too often considered normal effects of aging and can be treated.

Mild Cognitive Impairment: A Subtle Loss

A much milder version of thinking problems, called, appropriately, mild cognitive impairment (MCI), generally causes a smaller loss of brain function. It doesn't include personality changes, doesn't always progress to dementia, and isn't always due to Alzheimer's disease.

But MCI can often progress to Alzheimer's and is much more widespread than previously thought, especially in industrialized nations. A six-country report from the July 2011 Alzheimer's Association International Conference suggests that MCI affects between 15.4 and 42 percent of the populations that were studied and that between 8 and 15 percent of these progress to dementia each year.

High among the common factors that indicated the likely progression to Alzheimer's disease were mental attitudes and issues such as depression, apathy, and anxiety. Also important were age, low levels of education, loss of ability in activities of daily living, and cardiovascular factors such as stroke and diabetes.

In the U.S. portion of the study, the risk of progression was especially high for people who had stroke, depression, and several coexisting medical conditions. Other countries reported similar data. In Sweden, for example, diabetes accelerated the progression from MCI to dementia by three years.

Early treatment of these health issues, such as high blood pressure, high cholesterol, and diabetes, as well as depression, apathy, and anxiety, could slow or prevent progression of MCI, the researchers said.

The usual problems with MCI are trouble remembering names of new, recently met people; misplacing or forgetting items; and perhaps losing the flow of a conversation. People with MCI are often quite aware of the memory problems and develop ways to compensate for lapses with lists, calendars, and other reminders.

In many cases, the condition doesn't develop into dementia, but in some cases it will: people will develop problems performing daily activities, and the condition may progress to Alzheimer's or other dementia.

Encouragingly, very recent research is suggesting that MCI may be slowed, halted, or even partially reversed through exercise and lifestyle practices. (See Part Three, "How to Optimize Your Aging Brain.")

Stroke: The Brain Attack

Stroke ranks as the number four most common cause of death (behind heart disease, cancer, and chronic lower respiratory disease) but number one as the cause of disability and a contributor to dementia. The risk increases with age: nearly three-quarters of strokes occur after age 65, with the risk more than doubling each decade after age of 55.

Stroke does its damage by depriving the brain of oxygen through a blood clot (ischemic, which accounts for 87 percent of strokes) or a bleed (hemorrhagic, much less common, causes 7 to 10 percent). Sometimes a person can have a series of small strokes that increase the risk of a major stroke and lead to cumulative brain damage, so even very short-lasting symptoms call for immediate medical attention.

Getting treatment for an ischemic stroke within three hours of the onset of symptoms with tissue plasminogen activator (tPA) can dissolve clots and can often lessen disability if it is administered within three hours of an ischemic stroke. A hemorrhagic stroke caused when a blood vessel breaks and bleeds into the brain is much harder to treat: more than half are fatal.

But the prognosis for recovery is getting better as research reveals more effective poststroke therapies. Ten percent of stroke victims recover almost completely, and 25 percent recover with minor impairments. We used to give up too soon: doctors thought that the functions regained after three months were as good as it was going to get. Now we know that extending therapy may restore much more function.

COMING TO GRIPS WITH SLIPPAGE

If you do feel you may be losing your edge—if, for example, some mental activities seem to be becoming more difficult for you—it's a good idea to check things out medically. It could be what you are experiencing is normal aging, or it could be you need some help.

Here is what experts suggest to do if you see signs of a fading brain in yourself or someone else:

- *Get a workup and analysis.* This means a complete physical to see what's going on with your body, and perhaps an evaluation at a memory clinic to see what might be going on in your head. A geriatrician who specializes in issues of aging can help. Ask your primary care doctor for a referral.
- *Get a review of your current medications.* Ask your primary care doctor for an annual assessment. Some may be redundant, others outdated or even unneeded. Overmedication is a common contributor to mental confusion.
- *Ask your primary care doctor about counseling or therapy.* It could be some emotional issues are troubling you and causing some symptoms of mental lapses. And if you are having some memory issues and trouble with daily functioning, therapy can help you deal with what's happening.
- *Continue to socialize.* Don't let fear or anxiety isolate you. Talk to family and close friends about your feelings. Keep up relationships, and consider joining an activity group.
- *Consider increasing—or starting—physical and mental exercise.* Both are proven to help cognition and perhaps stop or slow mild cognitive impairment issues. Walking can be done at any time and anywhere. Your health maintenance organization, local health clinic, or senior center may have yoga, tai chi, and senior exercise programs.

Intensive therapy can help rewire a brain so that undamaged parts take up the slack from injured sections.

Stoke risk increases with the years but can strike at any age. Among the celebrities who have survived strokes and returned to active lives and their age at time of the stroke are Winston Churchill, 75; Academy award winner Patricia Neal, 39; *American Bandstand* host Dick Clark, 75; singer Brett Michaels, 47; and actors Sharon Stone, 43, Della Reese, 48, Kirk Douglas, 80, James Garner, 80, and Robert Guillaume, 72.

The same factors that contribute to dementia are also risks for stroke, so you may lower your risks of both with the same precautions. High blood pressure, for example, is the highest risk factor for stroke, and smoking doubles the risk for ischemic stroke and causes up to a fourfold increase in the risk of hemorrhagic stroke. Both are associated with dementia.

Lifestyle factors and medications can greatly reduce the risks: stroke risk decreases significantly two years after quitting smoking and is at the level of nonsmokers, and blood pressure medication reduces stroke risk by 30 to 40 percent.

Extensive physical therapy for many months helps many regain function. Recently, playing vigorous video games, such as the virtual reality sports of Wii, has been shown to help people recover both fine and gross motor function after stroke.

A Healing Stroke

Modern drugs swiftly applied lower brain damage from ischemic strokes. But researchers recently found a healing touch might work as well: tickling a rat's whiskers after it has a stroke prevents brain damage.

A team of neuroscientists stumbled on this very low-tech way to completely prevent stroke damage in rats. A team led by Professor Ron Frostig of the University of California, Irvine, induced strokes in rats

KNOWING THE SIGNS OF A STROKE

Damage from a stroke can be minimized if you act quickly, so if you experience these sudden signs or see them in someone else, call 911 immediately:

- Sudden numbness or weakness of the face, arm, or leg (especially on one side of the body)
- Sudden confusion or difficulty understanding speech
- Sudden loss of the ability to speak
- Sudden trouble seeing in one or both eyes
- Sudden trouble walking, dizziness, or loss of balance or coordination
- Sudden severe headache with no known cause

by blocking an artery to the brain. Then researchers stimulated their whiskers, intending to measure the rats' brain activity to learn how the stroke damage affected sensory functions. Instead they found that if they vibrated a single whisker within two hours of the stroke, neurons that ordinarily would have died continued to function normally, and the rats ended up with no paralysis or sensory deficits.

They don't know exactly why, but the touch seemed to involve a rerouting of blood through undamaged veins in the brain. Follow-up research published in the journal *Stroke* showed that the pattern of tickling does not matter (though more helps), and ongoing research in Frostig's lab has shown that the stimulation does not have to be tactile either. Auditory beeps prevented damage equally well.

The implications for human stroke victims are exciting, but there is no guarantee that playing music or touching sensitive areas such as the hands or face will have the same effect in people. It could be that the rat's much smaller brain might have helped their recovery. Still, Frostig is cautiously optimistic: "You may be able to help people way before the ambulance arrives, way before they can get any other treatment." It wouldn't hurt to talk to them and give their hands a squeeze on the way to the hospital, he says.

Parkinson's Disease

Parkinson's disease is due to a gradual degeneration of the brain cells that produce dopamine, the neurotransmitter that helps control voluntary movement. It's not generally fatal, usually comes on after age 60, and progresses slowly and gradually over years in most people. Approximately 1 million people in the United States are living with Parkinson's, many for twenty years or more, and prognosis varies greatly. With treatment, some people have a good quality of life for some years.

Parkinson's is believed to be caused by a combination of genetic and environmental factors. Genes account for 4 to 6 percent of Parkinson's, which may also be sparked by viruses or exposure to toxins such as pesticides. Brain injury may lead to dementia symptoms, as in the case of boxing great Muhammad Ali. The risk increases with age: the risk doubles from 1 to 2 percent to 2 to 4 percent after age 60, but it can attack much earlier. The actor Michael J. Fox developed Parkinson's disease in his 30s. He has been an active and prominent supporter of research.

There's no prevention or cure, but symptoms can be helped with medication. The development thirty years ago of levadopa, also known as l-dopa, was a major medical advance: it's converted to dopamine in the brain and is the primary treatment for Parkinson's disease, along with other medications. Innovative surgery in which battery-controlled electrodes are implanted to stimulate the brain (called deep brain stimulation, DBS) can dramatically help many people control tremors. Worldwide, about thirty thousand people have had DBS.

Recently scientists discovered that avid coffee drinkers and smokers have a lower risk of Parkinson's disease. To discover why, scientists at the University of Washington studied fruit flies that had been genetically engineered to have their dopamine cells die off as they age.

When the flies were fed coffee and tobacco extracts, their dopamine cells survived and their life span increased. Now, these may not be as protective as this seems: the scientists ruled out caffeine and nicotine as the protective substances. They are looking into other promising compounds in coffee and tobacco.

An intriguing preliminary small study that involved forced vigorous exercise (bicycling) has helped some people with Parkinson's improve symptoms. The study author, Jay L. Alberts, reports that people who biked for hour-long sessions over eight weeks on tandem bikes at a strenuous level regained some overall motor control. While it's not a cure, forced exercise could help retain or regain some waning functions.

Among those Parkinson's has struck are boxing great Muhammad Ali (born 1942), evangelist Billy Graham (born 1918), former U.S. attorney general Janet Reno (born 1938), Salvador Dalì (1904–1989), Pope John Paul II (1920–2005), president of Fiji Josefa Iloila (1920–2011), and film critic Pauline Kael (1919–2001).

Your Brain on Diabetes: Not So Sweet

Diabetes is a serious and potentially deadly disease. Anyone who has diabetes—or knows someone who has the disease—recognizes the importance of insulin, a hormone that helps cells store sugar and fat for energy; when the body can't produce enough of it (type 1 diabetes) or responds inadequately to it (type 2 diabetes), a range of circulatory and heart problems develops. And that's not all: research suggests that insulin is crucial for the brain, and insulin abnormalities have been implicated in a range of neurodegenerative diseases, including Alzheimer's and Parkinson's. Diabetes could contribute to dementia in several ways: insulin resistance may interfere with the body's ability to break down the toxic protein beta-amyloid that forms brain plaques, and high blood sugar (glucose) produces molecules that can damage cells by oxidative stress.

The risks for type 2 diabetes increase with age, with some ethnic groups, including African Americans, at higher risk than others. Other risk factors are similar to those that raise the risk of dementia, including inactivity, being overweight or obese, and having high blood pressure, high LDL (the "bad") cholesterol, and low HDL (the "good") cholesterol.

Historically, scientists believed that insulin was produced only by the pancreas and was not found in the central nervous system. Then in the mid-1980s, several research groups spotted the hormone and its receptor in the brain. It appeared that it not only crossed the blood-brain barrier but was also produced, at low levels, by the brain itself.

Soon afterward, scientists discovered that insulin plays an important role in learning and memory. People in research studies who inject or snort insulin immediately get better at recalling stories and performing other memory tasks. Conversely, learning raises insulin levels: rats mastering spatial memory tasks have higher brain insulin levels than sedentary rats do.

These observations led neuropathologist Suzanne de la Monte and her colleagues at Brown University to ask whether brain insulin might have a part in Alzheimer's disease. They compared insulin and insulin receptor levels in autopsies of healthy brains and brains of Alzheimer's disease patients. Average insulin levels in the neural areas associated with learning and memory were up to four times higher in the healthy brains, which also had up to ten times as many insulin receptors.

She refers to Alzheimer's disease as "type 3 diabetes." Because brain insulin is linked to insulin in the rest of the body through the blood-brain barrier, those with diabetes are more likely to develop

Alzheimer's disease too—nearly twice as likely, according to a 2002 study. They also suffer more memory and learning problems than the general population.

Researchers have found links between Alzheimer's disease and low brain levels of insulin-like growth factor 1 (IGF-1) and its receptor—proteins similar in structure to insulin and its receptor (insulin occasionally binds to the IGF-1 receptor, and vice versa). Some speculate that Alzheimer's disease is related to a loss of IGF to support brain cells and that defects in both insulin and IGF-1 could hurt the brain but they do not yet understand exactly how this works. Studies have also linked insulin and IGF-1 to Parkinson's disease: at least half of Parkinson's patients have glucose metabolism problems.

Some scientists believe that insulin is involved in the production of the large protein deposits similar to those seen in the brains of people with Alzheimer's and Parkinson's diseases. Although no one yet knows all the details, it appears that insulin and IGF-1 are crucial players in neurodegenerative disease.

Many scientists are working on potential treatments that restore normal insulin function in the hopes of easing or preventing neuro-degeneration: improved insulin response in the brain and body has been shown to lessen cognitive decline in early-stage Alzheimer's disease. Meanwhile, you might lower your risks of type 2 diabetes and its effects with some lifestyle practices. (See Part Three, "How to Optimize Your Aging Brain.")

Traumatic Brain Injury: A Blow to Your Thinking Brain

Traumatic brain injury (TBI) is among the major causes of brain damage, and in older folks it's not usually from an accident or being shot in the head, but rather from taking a fall.

A fall that injures the brain and other blows to the head are serious contributors to brain damage and a risk that increases with age: one out of three people over age 65 falls each year. People 75 years of age and older have the highest rates of TBI-related hospitalizations and death.

These tumbles often lead to an extended hospital stay, mark the move to an assisted living facility, and signal the downward spiral to death. "Given their frequency and consequences, falls are as serious a health problem for older persons as heart attacks or strokes," said Mary Tinetti of the Yale School of Medicine's Program in Geriatrics.

The Centers for Disease Control regards falls as a major health threat and recommends exercise to improve balance. (For ways to lower your risks of falling, see "A Fine Balance: Yoga, Tai Chi, and Fall Prevention" in Chapter Seven.) The Yale Program in Geriatrics also recommends reducing medications (if possible), avoiding alcohol, and increasing vitamin D.

Blows to the head over the years from other sources, including military combat, car accidents, and sports such as football, boxing, and ice hockey, are known to contribute to dementia. The Center for the Study of Traumatic Encephalopathy at the Boston University School of Medicine has found that imaging and analysis of the brains of some professional athletes who have had multiple concussions show extensive damage, even at a young age. So it's important for all of us to protect the head by wearing seat belts and using helmets for sports that could involve a fall, such as biking and skiing.

Depression: An Abnormal State

Depression is not a normal part of aging, but so many people believe it is that even severe depression goes undiagnosed and untreated in an estimated 50 percent of elders. Ironically, older folks often share the belief that depression is common and don't seek medical treatment because they think it won't help. That mistaken belief may prevent patients, their families, and even their doctors from checking into the many conditions or situations that can contribute to what looks like mental illness and can be treated. Still others with depression are victims of the opposite situation: they are overmedicated, which leads to more depression and sometimes symptoms of dementia. (See "Too Much of a Good Thing" later in this chapter.)

The truth is that depression rates, even with underreporting, are actually lower in healthy elders than in the general population, but elders do become more at risk as they face major life changes and losses, including deaths of a mate and friends and illness. Depression rates for people 65 and older jump from under 5 percent to 13.5 percent for those who require home health care.

Their doctors may fail to detect mental health issues because older patients often have multiple physical conditions, some quite serious. In fact, a study featured in the *Journal of the American Geriatrics Society* found that primary care doctors spend little time discussing mental health issues with older patients and that they rarely refer them to a mental health specialist even when patients show symptoms of severe depression. When a patient mentioned a mental health issue, as 22 percent did in the study, the discussion took only two minutes of the average sixteen-minute consultation.

Yet ignoring mental illness and depression in the elderly can indeed be life threatening. The Centers for Disease Control found in 2010 that while people age 65 and older represent 13 percent of the U.S. population, they accounted for 16 percent of suicide deaths and that men aged 75 and older made up 36.1 percent. The suicide rate in the overall population is 11.26 percent.

Studies have found that many older adults who commit suicide have visited a primary care physician very close to the time of the suicide: 20 percent on the same day and 40 percent within one week of the suicide.

WHEN DEPRESSION NEEDS TREATMENT

Feeling sadness and loss with aging is normal, and after a period of mourning, older people usually adjust and regain their emotional balance. But if you (or a loved one) have several of these signs of clinical depression, it's important to see a doctor:

- Persistent sadness lasting two or more weeks
- Withdrawing from regular social activities
- An empty feeling, ongoing sadness, and anxiety
- Fatigue, lack of energy
- Loss of interest or pleasure in everyday activities, including sex
- Sleep problems
- Eating more or less than usual
- Aches and pains that don't go away when treated
- A hard time focusing, remembering, or making decisions
- Feeling guilty, helpless, worthless, or hopeless
- Being irritable or frequent tearfulness
- Excessive worries about finances and health problems
- Pacing and fidgeting
- Weight or other appearance changes
- Thoughts of death or suicide or a suicide attempt

Depression has also been found to be a major contributor to MCI and a possible precursor to Alzheimer's disease. Severe depression may call for serious medications, but much depression in elders responds to a combination of mild antidepressants and some form of talk therapy, geriatricians say. Many elders don't want to be seen as complaining to their friends or children. Having a nonjudgmental listener helps evaluate fears and process feelings of sadness. Socializing can also help because loneliness contributes to depression.

The Legacy of Cancer: "Chemo Brain"

It doesn't seem fair: those who have endured and survived the rigors of cancer and cancer therapy often talk about memory and concentration problems they call "chemo brain."

Unfortunately, they're right. Research shows that people with a history of cancer have a 40 percent greater likelihood of having memory problems that interfere with daily functioning compared with those who have not had cancer. Researchers don't know why. The lifesaving cancer treatments of radiation and chemotherapy may cost patients their neurons and cause brain fogginess, or it could be other treatments or something in the cancer itself.

Researchers led by neurologist Michelle L. Monje of Harvard University have found one root of these cognitive difficulties: the chemicals and radiation used to kill tumor cells damaged stem cells in the hippocampus, a brain region vital for laying down new memories, and nearly halted the formation of new neurons in both children and adults.

Radiation treatment also triggers an inflammatory response from microglial cells, the immune cells of the central nervous system, and other experts think that the microglia may be the real culprit behind radiation-induced brain defects. Inflammation contributes to cognitive problems, and the researchers' previous work in rats showed that anti-inflammatory drugs helped to restore some neurogenesis.

A recent review of nearly ten thousand people found 14 percent of the thirteen hundred who had cancer reported memory problems compared to 8 percent who didn't have cancer, and that those with cancer were 40 percent more likely to have memory issues that interfered with daily functioning.

There's hope: exercise has been shown to stimulate neurogenesis in healthy animals and in people. Monje thinks there is a good chance that being active would help improve cognition in cancer survivors too.

Too Much of a Good Thing: When Medications Mess Up Your Mind

Could something your doctor ordered for you in good faith contribute to cognitive problems? Unfortunately, yes, at any age—but especially if you are an older American who may be taking multiple prescription, over-the-counter drugs, and herbal and other supplements.

Interactions, overdosing, and just plain wrong medications, including those prescribed and those sold over the counter, can be bad for your health and contribute to dementia-like symptoms. Many older people see multiple doctors who may not communicate with each other on their care of a particular patient and thus aren't aware of all the different medications their patients are taking—from five to fifteen or more. And when these are combined, they can have additive and toxic effects. One recent study found that older adults use 34 percent of all prescription medications, and many of these can provoke or mimic dementia symptoms.

Occasionally routine medications can create difficulties. Women who have trouble sleeping during their menopausal years may begin using sleeping pills and continue to use them for years. As they age, it can take longer for the active substance to dissipate in the body after waking, causing general drowsiness that complicates recall.

Or it could be an individual bad reaction to a single, well-regarded, and widely used drug. When 68-year-old Duane Graveline, a former astronaut, returned home from his morning walk in Merritt Island, Florida, he couldn't remember where he was and greeted his wife as a stranger. Six hours later in a hospital, when Graveline's memory returned, he wracked his brain to figure out what might have caused this terrifying bout of amnesia and confusion. Only one thing came to mind: he had recently started taking the statin drug Lipitor. As it turned out, he was one of the 5 percent who have a reaction to statins, a class of cholesterol-lowering drugs.

Lipitor and other cholesterol-lowering statins such as Crestor and Zocor are the most widely prescribed medications in the world, and they are credited with saving the lives of many with heart disease. But a small number of users have reported unexpected cognitive side effects such as Graveline's, including memory loss, fuzzy thinking, and learning difficulties. Hundreds have registered complaints with MedWatch, the U.S. Food and Drug Administration's adverse drug reaction database. For many, the benefits that statins provide overshadow the risks, but as with all other drugs, it's important to be aware of side effects.

Such symptoms, and even misdiagnoses, are more common as primary care doctors not trained in geriatrics treat a burgeoning caseload of older patients and tend to conclude many such symptoms are signs of dementia or, worse, a normal part of aging. Add to that a confused older person who doesn't have a relative or friend to advocate for him or her, and this person might not get needed treatment or could get treatment that could make symptoms worse.

It's also possible that someone may be taking medications no longer needed or duplicated. A long-term relationship with the same primary care doctor could help avert a misdiagnosis (or nondiagnosis) because that provider knows the patient. In addition, using the same pharmacy can be a safeguard against overmedication or drug interactions, and electronic record keeping may help keep prescriptions organized. But these days we tend to move around to be near children, grandchildren, and other loved ones, leaving behind the health care system where we (and our health conditions) are known.

Some medications may contribute to cognitive decline by interfering with your brain's ability to use acetylcholine, a neurotransmitter essential for good brain function. These are called anticholinergic agents, and you probably have a bunch of them in your medicine cabinet right now, in prescription or over-the-counter drugs as varied as antihistamines, antidepressants, antipsychotics, and some drugs used for urinary incontinence. The effects may be especially strong when two or more are taken in combination and can range from mild confusion to delirium.

YOUR FATTY BRAIN

When you think about it, it isn't crazy to connect cholesterol-modifying drugs with cognition. Cholesterol may be bad for your arteries, but it's vital for your brain: one-quarter of the body's cholesterol is found in the brain.

Cholesterol is a waxy substance that, among other things, provides structure to the body's cell membranes. High levels of cholesterol in the blood are not good: they create a risk for heart disease because the molecules that transport cholesterol can damage arteries and cause blockages. But in the brain, cholesterol plays a crucial role in forming neuronal connections—the vital links among brain cells that underlie memory and learning. Quick thinking and rapid reaction times depend on cholesterol, the building blocks of the sheaths that insulate your neurons and speed up electrical transmissions. So it makes sense that a drug that affects such an important pathway could have adverse reactions.

The evidence is not conclusive. A link between statins and cognitive problems was suggested in two small trials published in 2000 and 2004, and a 2003 study published in *Reviews of Therapeutics* noted that among sixty statin users who had reported memory problems to MedWatch, more than half said their symptoms improved when they stopped taking the drugs.

But other studies have found no significant link between statins and memory problems, and some even suggest that statins might improve memory in certain people by lowering the risk of dementia, since cholesterol is involved in the production of the protein clusters that are the hallmark of neurodegenerative diseases such as Alzheimer's and Parkinson's diseases. Simply switching statin drugs might help people who are experiencing warning signs such as forgetting names.

Talk to your doctor about using the medications listed here: the benefit might outweigh any risks. And of course, be sure to consult with your doctor before stopping any prescription medication.

Allergy and cold drugs and ingredients are ubiquitous and often anticholinergic. One, diphenhydramine (better known as Benadryl), is in many combination cold drugs and often used as a sleep aid. Others are chlorpheniramine, sold as Chlortrimeton, and pseudo-ephedrine, an ingredient in many allergy meds.

Drugs for depression that interfere with acetylcholine include the tricyclic antidepressants such as amitriptyline (Elavil), trazadone (Desyryl), nortriptyline (Pamelor), and imipramine (Tofranil). Some nursing homes and doctors hand out powerful antipsychotics such as thorazine and clozapine to elders who express distress, both to ease their discomfort but also to quiet them down. These are also anticholinergics.

Other widely used medications are suspected anticholinergics. The list is long and includes the diuretic Lasix (furosemide); digoxin, a form of digitalis used for heart conditions; theophyline, prescribed for asthma and other lung conditions; prednisolone, a corticosteroid steroid used to reduce inflammation; codeine; nifedipine, a calcium-channel blocker used to treat high blood pressure; cimetidine (Tagamet) and ranitidine (Zantac), used to treat ulcers and gastroesophageal reflux disease; and coumadin (Warfarin), one of the most widely used of all drugs, to prevent blood clots. For more information and a list of on anticholinergic drugs, go to http://www.indydiscoverynetwork .org/AnticholienrgicCognitiveBurdenScale.html.

What—Me Worry?

It would be surprising if this catalogue of brain diseases and disasters didn't produce a twinge of concern. It's never very pleasant to contemplate potential problems. And there are many unknowns that can add to the concern. We don't know enough yet about the brain to be able to predict with certainty and with a few exceptions who will succumb to any of these conditions and who will escape.

There are some things you can do that might lower your risks of some brain conditions. It would help, in some cases, to have chosen better genetic material in your ancestors or perhaps to refuse to age, but neither of these is possible.

Part Three distills the current research on what experts believe you can do to optimize your brain health. The usual items top the list: not smoking, exercising, maintaining a healthy weight, eating well, and avoiding stress. Although these practices are no guarantee for longer life, they may help you to live and feel better in the here and now.

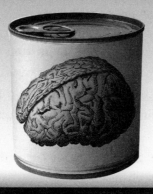

CHAPTER FIVE

Alzheimer's Disease

The Brain Killer

It's the 800-pound gorilla, the elephant in the living room: the terrifying yet often unspoken possibility of losing your mind as your brain ages.

Alzheimer's and other dementias are among the greatest health fears worldwide, second only to cancer. In fact, Alzheimer's may be the most significant social and health crisis of the twenty-first century, according to the Alzheimer's Disease International 2011 "World Alzheimer Report."

And no wonder: it comes with extraordinary personal, emotional, and economic costs. It's devastating to lose your memories and yourself in the fog of brain cell death and for your loved ones to lose you. The cost of care does more than cripple individuals and families: it takes a huge social toll, and the economic cost is nearly as staggering.

Millions have the disease, and tens of millions more will be affected directly and indirectly in caring for loved ones. So far, in spite of billions spent on research, there is no effective treatment, no cure, and not even a definitive understanding of what causes this brain-killing disease.

Researchers are getting closer to determining the causes of Alzheimer's. They know that it causes loss of mental functions by destroying the connections among brain cells and then the neurons themselves. They have found what may be the footprints of dementia in sticky tangles in the brain, plaques, and atrophy of brain tissue. They have also identified some genetic connections. But they aren't certain if the brain gunk is a cause or an effect of Alzheimer's or how and why the disease hits some of us and not others. Genes are a direct cause of only a tiny number of Alzheimer's cases—probably less than 1 percent. There are several genes known to raise one's risk of getting the disease, but by how much, and why, isn't known yet.

Studies are increasingly connecting an unhealthy lifestyle with dementia. Those with known risks fall prey—but then so do those who have led exemplary healthy lives and appear to have no genetic connection, while others with unhealthy life practices seem to be unscathed. Alzheimer's is indiscriminate, affecting former presidents, sports heroes, movie and rock stars, literary giants, and, increasingly, fictional characters in films, television, and books as the inexorable wave of this disease becomes part of our culture.

What Is Alzheimer's Disease?

Dementia comes in many guises, can be caused by many diseases and conditions, and varies widely in its onset and initial effects. It's characterized by a loss of memory and thinking skills, interferes with the ability to make decisions, and eventually takes away the ability to participate in the most basic activities.

Alzheimer's is by far the most common kind of dementia, accounting for up to 80 percent of cases. It's a progressive condition most known for causing memory loss and, eventually, death.

Alzheimer's and other dementias often start with a condition called mild cognitive impairment (MCI), which is characterized by memory and thinking problems greater than those associated with normal aging but not severe enough to disrupt daily life. People with MCI generally don't show the personality changes found in Alzheimer's, and not everyone with MCI develops Alzheimer's. Some do go on to develop other types of dementia or neurological conditions, while others remain stable for years. Studies are showing that some life practices, such as increased exercise and improved nutrition, may prevent, reverse, or keep MCI from progressing to dementia. (See Part Three, "How to Optimize Your Aging Brain.")

Early diagnosis is important, but it is difficult because, researchers believe, the disease starts as long as twenty years before symptoms appear. So far, scientists will say (with rather brutal frankness) that the only 100 percent accurate diagnosis of Alzheimer's is a brain autopsy. However, doctors skilled in working with dementia can make an accurate diagnosis 80 to 90 percent of the time. Several types of tests can find early signs of the disease. Levels of brain-damaging proteins called beta-amyloid and tau can be detected by taking a sample of cerebrospinal fluid (CSF) in what is called a spinal tap. The less amyloid in the CSF, the more of it is likely to be in the brain and the greater the likelihood is that the person has Alzheimer's. In contrast, having more tau protein in the CSF is correlated with a higher risk. This test is invasive and not widely used. Imaging scans can show Alzheimer's damage in the brain and shrinkage in brain volume after the disease has progressed.

But here's another conundrum: even a brain ravaged by such damage may function adequately. Autopsies of the brains of seemingly normal people—people who functioned quite well in life—have found signs of extensive Alzheimer's-type changes.

SOME FACTS ABOUT ALZHEIMER'S DISEASE

Alzheimer's disease was first described in 1906 by Alois Alzheimer, the German physician it's named for, when he discovered abnormal clumps and fiber tangles in the brain of a woman who died in her 50s of what was then an unusual mental illness. Relatively unnoticed for decades, Alzheimer's became considered a serious issue about thirty years ago. Today it is of international concern.

- Alzheimer's disease is marked by a progressive loss of cognitive and physical function, ending in death.
- Two telltale signs of Alzheimer's are clumps of sticky gunk in the brain called beta-amyloid plaques, and neurofibrillary tangles made of an abnormal form of a protein called tau. Scientists believe that these lesions destroy connections among neurons and eventually cause brain cell death. Over the course of the disease, parts of the brain involved in thinking and memory, especially the cortex and hippocampus, deteriorate markedly.
- Brain changes leading to Alzheimer's begin as many as ten to twenty years before any obvious outward signs. By the time there are symptoms, the brain cells that process, store, and retrieve information have already begun to degenerate and die.
- There is currently no cure and no truly effective treatment for Alzheimer's. Researchers aren't even sure of the cause.
- One in eight Americans older than 65 (about 13 percent) have Alzheimer's, or about 5.4 million people. Nearly 44 percent of those over age 85 have the disease. Two-thirds of those (3.4 million) are women, who generally live longer than men.
- Worldwide, more than 35 million people have dementia, much of it caused by Alzheimer's disease, a figure projected to nearly double to 66 million by 2030.
- Alzheimer's disease is the fifth leading cause of death in the United States for those older than 65.
- Most people survive an average of four to eight years after an Alzheimer's diagnosis, but some live as long as twenty years. On average, 40 percent of those years are spent in the most severe stage of the disease, longer than any other stage.
- Four percent of the general population will be admitted to a nursing home by age 80. But 75 percent of people with Alzheimer's will be in a nursing home by that age.

Chasing the Cause

Intensive research has identified some factors that contribute to or increase the risk of dementia, but scientists don't have all the answers yet. In fact, the theories, research, and contributing factors range widely.

Although accumulation of the proteins beta-amyloid and tau is among the brain changes believed to contribute to Alzheimer's disease, researchers aren't sure if this is a cause or an effect. Genetics plays a role, but apparently in connection with environmental and other factors, and researchers don't yet understand how important it may be.

A small percentage of Alzheimer cases—fewer than 1 percent—is caused by rare genetic variations that virtually guarantee the disease before age 65, sometimes in individuals as young as 30 years old. Called familial Alzheimer's, this is found in only a few hundred families worldwide. It involves the gene for the amyloid precursor protein on chromosome 21, the gene for the presenilin 1 protein on chromosome 14, and the gene for the presenilin 2 protein on chromosome 1. Having at least one first-degree relative with dementia seems to double or quadruple the lifetime risk of developing Alzheimer's, but researchers have not found a specific gene for the more prevalent late-onset form of the disease. One genetic risk factor does appear to increase a chance of developing the disease later in life: ApoE4, a version of the apoliprotein E (Apoe) gene. It's quite common, found in about 25 percent of all of us and in 40 percent of all people with late-onset Alzheimer's disease, and having more than one copy of this gene seems to increase the risk. But having this form of the gene doesn't mean you'll get the disease: some people even inherit two copies of the gene and don't get it; others have none and still develop it. To make it more confusing, different forms of apoliprotein seem to affect beta-amyloid and inflammatory response differently: the ApoE3 form is neutral, and another version, ApoE2, the least common version, seems to lower Alzheimer's risk, and researchers are discovering several other so-called risk genes, but they don't seem as strong.

Some good news: the increased genetic risk decreases with age. So if you make it into your 80s without getting Alzheimer's, having a first-degree relative with the disease may not matter so much.

In fact, as scientists learn more, they've come to realize that genetics alone rarely dictates the course of most brain disorders. As with other conditions, most neurological disorders are the result of a complex interaction between genes and environment, perhaps triggered by multiple processes, and will need more than one type of treatment. Therefore, genetic testing may not be useful until its role is better understood, unless there is a very strong family connection with early-onset familial Alzheimer's that suggests the presence of the three rare definitive gene variants. Also, blood tests can tell if one carries the alipoprotein genes, for example, but these genes are so common that their presence can't predict who will develop Alzheimer's disease. It's not certain genetic testing will ever be able to predict the disease with 100 percent accuracy in most cases because too many other factors may influence its development and progression, just as in other diseases. For example, people can inherit the tendency for high blood pressure and high cholesterol, two well-established risk factors for heart disease, and still not have a heart attack.

You may not want to know if you have an elevated genetic risk. James Watson, one of the scientists who discovered DNA, didn't: he had his APOE gene "blacked out" when he had his genome sequenced a couple years ago.

However, if you do have Alzheimer's in your family, you may want to enroll in the national Alzheimer's Disease Genetics Study. Healthy volunteers over age 60 who have no neurological diseases or conditions are also needed. See the Resources section at the back of this book for information about the National Cell Repository for Alzheimer's Disease and other organizations.

CONNECTIONS AND CONSIDERATIONS

Increasing age is the major risk factor for Alzheimer's disease, and there's not much we can do about that. But we're learning more every day about other conditions and circumstances that may be linked with risk of developing dementia. Fortunately, many of these are situations or conditions you can change or control:

- Heart disease, stroke, and high blood pressure. Cardiovascular health is closely linked to brain health since blood flow nourishes and supports the brain.
- Chronic inflammation, which is related to many diseases and conditions and destroys neurons.
- Diabetes, which some studies suggest may as much as double Alzheimer's risk.
- Chronic depression, which studies show may double your risk of dementia.
- Anxiety and stress. Chronic stress makes the brains of experimental animals less resilient and seems to be connected in humans with a higher risk of memory loss and dementia.
- Physical and mental inactivity and obesity, which also increase heart disease risks.
- Smoking, which harms the cardiovascular system, raising the risks of stroke and dementia.
- Genetics, especially in combination with other factors, which contributes to risks of both early- and late-onset Alzheimer's, but scientists don't understand all the genes or risks involved yet.

Anxiety and Alzheimer's Disease: Another Reason to Chill

As research turns up more connections between lifestyle and dementia, evidence is mounting that a lifetime of emotional stress, such as anxiety or fear, could lead to memory problems and can make a person more susceptible to Alzheimer's.

Now, not all stress is bad. A bit of some occasional stress—amusement park rides, a horror movie, perhaps even bungee jumping—tunes us up and turns us on. But constant stress wears our bodies down like tires spinning on rock, and it's known to contribute to heart disease and other conditions.

Scientists have connected memory issues with stress in several animal studies and some observational studies of humans. They find that although stress alone doesn't degrade memory, it does seem to push at-risk animals over the edge, making them less able to learn and remember new things.

When a team at the Salk Institute for Biological Studies in San Diego induced mild stress in mice by physically restraining the animals for half an hour, they found the incident modified the tau protein, which gives neurons structural support, thereby rendering it unable to fulfill its role. The good news is that after a single stress episode, tau morphed back into its original state within ninety minutes. But when the team induced stress every day for two weeks, tau remained in its modified state long enough to allow individual protein molecules to clump together. These protein heaps are the first step toward neurofibrillary tangles, one of the hallmarks associated with Alzheimer's disease.

Other animal studies show that tight quarters cause stress in animals, elevating levels of glucocorticoid hormones in their blood. In humans, cortisol, a glucocorticoid hormone released by stress, influences a number of brain regions. When cortisol binds to a specialized molecular receptor, the interaction triggers events that reduce com-munication at synapses, the junctions between neurons, which may ultimately cause the connections to wither away.

Researchers have studied the brains of aged rhesus monkeys that had spent their early lives in either small or standard-size cages, using protein stains that adhere specifically to synapses. The team then determined the relative number of synapses in all the monkeys, as well as the amount of sticky amyloid plaques.

They found that the monkeys raised in the smaller cages had, on average, a significantly higher density of damaging plaques and fewer synapses in one part of their brain—the same pattern seen in the brains of Alzheimer's patients at autopsy. The finding suggested that stress could make a brain vulnerable as it ages. They noted a wide reaction to stress: the amount of plaque riddling the brains of the monkeys housed in smaller cages varied a lot, indicating that stress affects individuals differently. After all, we all know people who seem to take even mildly negative events to heart as well as others in similar situations who take their plight in stride.

A more recent study with rodents suggests that even intermittent strain can tip the scales toward dementia when combined with other risk factors. Neuropharmacologist Karim Alkadhi at the University of Houston and his colleagues put rats at risk for dementia by injecting them with very low concentrations of amyloid peptides, and then stressed some of the animals by placing an intruder rat in their home cage. As expected, the blood levels of corticosterone (a stress hormone related to cortisol) rose in the stressed rats.

Then the scientists placed each rat in a water tank, where they had to find the path that led to a platform to escape—a rodent test of learning and memory. Most of the experimental rats, including those that had been given amyloid injections and those forced to face intrud-ers, performed well. But the rats that had received both the shots and the unwanted visitor struggled.

Other animal research hints that stress may hasten the onset of Parkinson's disease as well. Behavioral neuroscientist Gerlinde A. S. Metz and her colleagues at the University of Lethbridge in Alberta created Parkinson's disease–like conditions in rats by infusing a toxic drug into a brain area rich with dopamine neurons. They then boosted stress hormones in some of the rats and discovered the ones with the double-whammy did not recover as fast as the ones with only dopamine damage, suggesting that stress might trigger or aggravate Parkinson's symptoms.

So far, the evidence is limited. Does this mean people who are prone to chronic worry and tension can have memory problems in old age? Perhaps.

A study by Robert Wilson and his colleagues at Rush University Medical Center in Chicago evaluated the stress susceptibility of more than one thousand elderly people by rating their agreement with statements such as, "I am often tense and jittery." They found that over a period of up to twelve years, volunteers who said they were anxiety prone had a 40 percent higher risk of developing mild cognitive impairment than their more easygoing counterparts did.

Mild cognitive impairment is thought to be a frequent precursor for Alzheimer's disease, but brain autopsies on study participants who died didn't show evidence of neurofibrillary tangles or any of the other known features indicative of Alzheimer's disease, Wilson says. Still, he thinks it is possible that chronic distress gradually compromises memory systems, ultimately leaving the brain vulnerable to the physical changes associated with Alzheimer's.

The good news here is that stress and anxiety are conditions that can be controlled with exercise, meditation, therapy, medications, and perhaps just getting enough sleep. These are yet more reasons to chill out and work out because these may help reduce the stress of life's encounters (see the chapters in Part Three, "How to Optimize Your Aging Brain").

Maybe It's Bad Neural Housekeeping?

Could Alzheimer's disease be connected, at least partly, to bad house-keeping in your brain?

Studies show that your body is constantly at work to vacuum up cellular debris that could gum up the works. Indeed, researchers are now wondering if dementia could be the result of a breakdown in your brain's self-cleaning system.

Every day and night, your body cleans up your neural garbage, removing damaged and dying cells in a process called autophagy (or "self-eating," from the Greek), much the way our bodies dispose of invading viruses and bacteria.

Autophagosomes clean up and digest the cytoplasm inside your cells where a vast and intricate array of complex operations produces what is basically trash. Proteins, for instance, which carry out the work of the cell, are sometimes put together wrong and can stop functioning or, worse, may malfunction. Autophagy cleans up the cytoplasm that's clotted with old bits of protein and other unwanted sludge made up of old and damaged cellular machinery.

When autophagy runs too slowly, too quickly, or otherwise malfunctions, the consequences can be dire indeed. Slovenly autophagy might play a pivotal role in Alzheimer's, Parkinson's, and other neurodegenerative disorders such as Huntington's disease. All of these brain diseases are characterized by clumps of defective proteins and other cellular trash that the cells fail to clear away. Some think this is evidence that autophagy is failing to do its job and suggest that a breakdown in autophagy may contribute to Alzheimer's disease.

One of the most frequent effects of normal aging is the accumulation of a brownish material called lipofuscin, a mix of lipids and proteins, in the bodies of brain cells. Superficially the stuff can be likened to liver spots on aging skin. The accumulation is a sign that aging brain cells can no longer remove abnormally

ALZHEIMER'S IS NOT INEVITABLE

Adapting to the inevitable losses of aging, including the deaths of mate and friends, may leave some people feeling temporarily confused or forgetful. But these are not usually signs of dementia. Alzheimer's, like any other dementia, is not a normal part of aging, even though the risks increase with age: it is a disease.

Among researchers' finding are these:

- Not everyone is at risk. Although nearly 45 percent of those over age 85 are estimated to have Alzheimer's disease, that is still not 100 percent, and some evidence holds that lifestyle practices may lower the risk.

- Genes are not destiny. A very small number of people who carry rare genetic mutations will inevitably develop Alzheimer's. But for most of us, heritable factors may increase risk (but by no means guarantee we will develop the disease), or could be protective and lower Alzheimer's risk. It appears that a combination of factors contributes to dementia.

- You may be able to lower your risk, and stop or reverse some of the effects of mild cognitive impairment, with lifestyle practices. Although there is no scientifically proven preventive, studies are showing that staying physically, mentally, and socially active and controlling weight, blood pressure, and diabetes are associated with a lower risk of developing dementia. Earlier is better, but it is never too late to start. (See the chapters in Part Three, "How to Optimize Your Aging Brain.")

- Alzheimer's affects everyone somewhat differently, and the severity varies. The onset may be abrupt, or it may evolve slowly. Some people adapt and function with limitations for many years. Only in the familial early-onset type do we know the inevitable outcome will arrive sooner rather than later.

- Not all brains succumb to Alzheimer's damage. Some people whose brains were autopsied after death showed signs of extensive Alzheimer's-type damage yet appeared normal and functioned quite well in life. Some suggest that cognitive reserve—the mental resiliency connected with higher levels of education and involvement in creative and social activities—may give some protection, but scientists don't actually know the reason.

With scientists worldwide focused on dementia research, it's likely that effective treatments to treat, prevent, or slow Alzheimer's will be discovered. Some scientists believe this could be within decades if enough resources are focused on research.

modified or damaged proteins fast enough to keep pace with their buildup.

In people with Alzheimer's, a yellowish or brownish pigment called ceroid also builds up inside neurites (projections from nerve cell bodies). The neurites swell where ceroid collects, and amyloid plaques form on the outside of the swollen neurites. So far investigators don't know the exact ways amyloid leads to neuron damage. But the latest research shows, tellingly, that enzymes that help to deposit the plaques in certain early-onset forms of Alzheimer's disease are present on the membranes of autophagosomes.

Given this, it would seem likely that promoting autophagy might slow the onset of the debilitating symptoms of Alzheimer's. A drug that does that is being tested for Huntington's, a devastating neurological disease that is genetic and fatal and characterized by protein clumps.

It could also be that taking out the neural trash plays a role in determining your life span, keeping your vital cells healthier and stronger longer. A good cleaning is particularly important to neurons because they are long lived—as long lived as you are in most cases. We take it for granted that many diseases become more frequent with age, including cancer and dementia. The reason, in part, may be a matter of failing housekeeping.

The Search for a Cure—or Even a Treatment That Works

Alzheimer's disease is the only one among the top ten causes of death in America without a way to prevent, cure, or even slow its progression. It's not for lack of trying. As the epidemic of dementia has been growing, billions have been spent worldwide on diagnosis and treatments, and scientists remain hard at work.

Any drug that could delay or stop Alzheimer's disease would be an immediate blockbuster. There are a few that may ease symptoms temporarily but no actual disease-modifying drugs on the market yet, largely because researchers are still trying to understand the underlying mechanisms of the disease.

Drugs that interfere with amyloid buildup offer a case in point. A number of drug possibilities at various stages of testing can purportedly inhibit amyloid accumulation or foster its clearance. Yet several antiamyloid drugs tested in clinical trials have so far failed, raising doubt whether limiting amyloid will benefit memory and thinking. It will almost certainly depend on when the drugs are administered. If they're administered too late, the damage is done and is unlikely to be reversed simply by clearing amyloid.

Amyloids produced in the brains of people with Alzheimer's do their damage by rapidly killing so-called cholinergic neurons, those that synthesize acetylcholine—the neurotransmitter that improves thinking mood, behavior, and overall daily functioning. Drugs called cholinesterase inhibitors increase levels of acetylcholine but are only moderately effective; the disease continues to progress and kill brain cells.

Only a few drugs have been approved by the U.S. Food and Drug Administration (FDA) and are on the market. One group of drugs called acetylcholinesterase inhibitors, such as donepezil (Aricept) and galantamine (Nivalin, Razadyne), block the action of the enzyme acetylcholinesterase and boost levels of acetylcholine.

Another drug called memantine (Namenda) is an NMDA (*N*-methyl *D*-aspartate) receptor antagonist, which helps quell overactivity from the signaling chemical glutamate that can lead to the death of neurons. But neither drug interferes with the buildup of cell lesions that may push progression of the disease. And to repeat, the drugs available in early 2012 treat cognitive symptoms only, not the underlying disease process, and they work only for a limited time, from months to a few years.

Many experts believe these drugs simply offer too little too late. Since much of the damage is under way well before memory loss becomes apparent, successful treatment must start during the many years before symptoms appear. By the time a doctor can make a diagnosis and prescribe medication, so many brain cells have been destroyed that boosting the amount of acetylcholine is as futile as sticking a bandage on a massive head wound.

They agree the best treatment would be early detection and prevention. Therefore, a major thrust of much Alzheimer's disease research is shifting toward catching and stopping the disease before symptoms show—not only with drugs but also with lifestyle measures that would be safer and less costly than filling a drug prescription for ten or twenty years. Recent research is suggesting that exercise, diet, and social and mental activity may substantially reduce Alzheimer's risks. (See the chapters in Part Three, "How to Optimize Your Aging Brain.")

A program called the Alzheimer's Prevention Initiative is planning trials in which healthy family members around the age of 40 who carry mutations for familial Alzheimer's disease would start to receive antiamyloid therapies (a drug or vaccine) already tested for safety in Alzheimer's patients. They are first planning to work with families in Medellín, Colombia, which has the largest contingent in the world of people with the lethal heritable form of familial Alzheimer's disease, invariably developing the disease before age 50. The trial would evaluate whether a treatment can delay or stop

PROMISING THERAPIES IN THE WORKS

There is financial as well as medical incentive for developing a drug that could substantively delay or stop Alzheimer's. Given the demographic bulge of baby boomers approaching old age, its sales would perhaps exceed those for Prozac or Lipitor. No such drugs are on the market because investigators are still trying to understand how to alter the underlying mechanisms that lead to brain death. As with cancer and HIV, it may be necessary to combine several of these agents to slow or halt Alzheimer's. The table lists major classes of Alzheimer's drugs under development.

One of the most prominent and promising treatments is immunotherapy: vaccines that either trigger the body's immune system to produce antibodies to attach the beta-amyloid or in some cases deliver the antibody directly to the amyloids. These therapies are still in the early stages, with ongoing clinical trials. They hold promise as a realistic therapy down the road, especially if people in the presymptomatic stage of the disease can be identified and get the vaccine before it is too late.

Drugs Types Under Study	What They Do
Inhibitors of enzymes that produce beta-amyloid	Such inhibitors block or modify the action of enzymes that cut a large protein (the amyloid precursor protein) in a way that releases the beta-amyloid peptides.
Vaccines or antibodies that clear beta-amyloid	Vaccines prompt the body to produce antibodies that bind to amyloid and clear them from the brain. Unfortunately, in clinical trials so far, both vaccines and antibodies have induced side effects of varying severity in some patients.
Beta-amyloid aggregation blockers	Agents that prevent amyloid fragments from clumping could prevent damage to neurons.

Drugs Types Under Study	What They Do
Anti-tau compounds	These agents, although fewer in number than those that target amyloids, take various approaches, such as blocking production of the toxic form of the tau protein or impeding its aggregation into tangles.
Neuroprotective agents	Different strategies attempt to boost natural brain chemicals that contribute to the health of neurons. In one, a gene is delivered into the brain to start production of a protective substance.

the inexorable silent progression of the disease if administered seven years before the average age of diagnosis in family members known to carry the gene.

Researchers also plan to see whether tracking Alzheimer's-specific biomarkers can indicate whether an experimental treatment is working. (A biomarker is a measurable indicator, such as a concentration of a particular protein, that changes in concert with progression or regression of a disease.) A reliable set of biomarkers would allow drug researchers and doctors caring for patients to evaluate the success of a therapy relatively quickly by measuring changes in such silent benchmarks instead of having to wait to assess overt symptoms, which may not show up until the disease has progressed.

And some researchers wonder whether too little emphasis has been placed on interfering with other processes that contribute to the disease. Among the one hundred or so agents under development are many drugs that target the cell-damaging beta-amyloid and tau protein, and also those that quell inflammation, boost the functioning of mitochondria, enhance cerebral insulin levels, or provide other protection for neurons.

Researchers are working on some exciting and novel therapies, including a chemical switch to manipulate genes, a vaccine, drugs to stop or reverse mental deterioration, and even computer chip brain implants to supplement memory. The Alzheimer Disease Neuroimaging Initiative, the largest Alzheimer's disease study ever funded by the National Institutes of Health and a coalition of industry and nonprofit organizations, has researchers at fifty-nine centers looking for ways to predict the onset of the disease.

Some researchers are also studying lifestyle changes and behaviors (such as exercise, diet, socializing, and mental activity) to see if and how they affect both who gets dementia and the progress of the disease (see Part Three, "How to Optimize Your Aging Brain").

Looking Beyond the Brain

Some researchers are looking beyond the brain for causes and contributors to Alzheimer's disease and at some drugs long used effectively for other conditions, including antirejection, cancer, epilepsy, and schizophrenia drugs.

Mitochondria, the components responsible for the energy regulation of cells, could be a missing link in the Alzheimer's puzzle. Researchers at Columbia University have found that young mice predisposed to developing Alzheimer's accumulate protein clusters in the mitochondria at their synapses—the tiny gaps between cells over which energy and information are passed to create networks vital for thinking. This directly interferes with synapse function and the communication of information between cells.

Studies have suggested that beta-amyloid proteins, the type found in Alzheimer's disease, interfere with mitochondria function. But no one knew exactly how mitochondria were linked to synaptic problems, if at all. To find out, Shirley ShiDu Yan and her colleagues at the Columbia University Medical Center genetically engineered mice to overproduce a compound that leads to the formation of destructive beta-amyloid clusters. Then, when the mice were at various ages, the researchers took mitochondria from regions near their synapses and from other brain regions. When the mice were just four months old, well before they showed symptoms of disease, the mitochondria in their synapses had accumulated approximately five times more amyloid protein than the mitochondria from other cells.

They found evidence that the damaged mitochondria couldn't give the synapses enough energy to function properly, providing the first direct link between cell injury caused by beta-amyloid protein and the breakdown of neural networks that is characteristic of Alzheimer's disease. In earlier research, Yan reported that cyclosporin D, a drug used to prevent organ transplant rejection and to treat autoimmune diseases, prevents beta-amyloid proteins from injuring mitochondria. Cyclosporin has serious side effects, so Yan is looking to develop a similar but safer compound to prevent synaptic problems early on.

The liver turns out to be another unexpected area for research and possible treatments. A recent study suggests that the liver, and not the brain, might be a larger source of beta-amyloid plaque than previously thought. Scientists working with a mouse model of Alzheimer's disease found three genes that protected mice from accumulating beta-amyloid in the brain and lower activity of each of these genes in the liver protected the mouse brain. One of the genes produces presenilin 2, a known contributor to beta-amyloid production. It was found in the liver of the mice but not in the brain, suggesting that some beta-amyloid might originate in the liver, circulate in the blood, and enter the brain. If this is correct, blocking liver production of beta-amyloid might help protect the brain.

In complex tests with mice, they found the cancer drug imatinib, an FDA-approved leukemia drug, dramatically reduced amyloid not only in the blood but also in the brain. This was remarkable because the blood-brain barrier prevents the drug from penetrating the brain. That suggests both that some brain beta-amyloid originates outside the brain and that the drug could be a candidate for treating Alzheimer's disease.

Research presented at the Alzheimer's Association 2011 International Conference also suggests that excess brain activity in patients with a condition known as amnestic mild cognitive impairment (aMCI) contributes to brain dysfunction that underlies memory loss. Previously it had been thought that this hyperactivity was the brain's attempt to "make up" for weakness in its ability to form new memories.

An epilepsy drug is showing some promise too. Levetiracetam, an anticonvulsant, is used in combination with other drugs to treat certain types of epileptic seizures. It's already approved for use in some aging epilepsy patients to slow abnormal loss of brain function. A Johns Hopkins University study found hyperactive brain activity in patients with aMCI. They studied older adults, some healthy and others with memory difficulties associated with aMCI, using functional magnetic resonance imaging to study brain activity during a memory task. Those with aMCI had extra activity in the hippocampus, but after taking levetiracetam for two weeks, the excess activity dropped to the same level as that of the healthy subjects.

Researchers are also looking at the schizophrenia drug lithium—and beyond. For example, consider marijuana.

An Ounce of Prevention: Marijuana Might Benefit Aging Brains

Clinton didn't inhale, Obama did—and maybe Reagan should have. New research suggests that tetrahydrocannabinol (THC), the chemical that gives marijuana its mind-bending properties, is very bad for young neurons, but it actually saves neurons in adults with Alzheimer's disease.

Marijuana is infamous for its ability to muddle thoughts and dull reactions, so who would have thought it might blunt the progression of Alzheimer's disease? Research reveals that the active ingredient in marijuana, THC, may outperform acetylcholinesterase inhibitors. In older brains, like the brains of boomers and beyond—the ones at risk of Alzheimer's—THC seems to have a protective effect.

This is puzzling because using marijuana during the period of life when the young brain is still developing messes up critical chemical signals, research suggests, and could explain the developmental cognitive impairment seen in children born to women who smoked marijuana during pregnancy. When neuropharmacologist Veronica Campbell of Trinity College in Dublin and her coworkers treated brain cells from newborn or adolescent rats with THC, the neurons died. But THC didn't have such deadly effects on neurons taken from adult rats.

Several possibilities are being investigated for this Jekyll and Hyde effect. Marijuana, like tobacco and opium, has powerful effects on the brain because certain compounds in the plant happen to have a chemical resemblance to substances that naturally occur in the body.

Campbell's findings suggest that the biochemistry of neurons changes as the cells mature. Endocannabinoids and cannabinoids, natural chemicals similar to those in marijuana, regulate important brain functions by controlling synapses in neural circuits that process thought and perception. Their role shifts to regulate different functions, including—most important—assisting in the survival of aged neurons. In those with Alzheimer's disease, THC protects neurons from death in several ways. It boosts depleted levels of the neurotransmitter acetylcholine, which, when diminished, contributes to the weakened mental function in Alzheimer's patients. THC also suppresses the toxic effects of the beta-amyloid protein that contributes to neuronal cell death in Alzheimer's disease, stimulates secretion of neuron growth by promoting substances such as brain-derived neuro-trophic factor, and dampens release of the excitatory neurotransmitter glutamate, which kills neurons by overstimulation. THC and other cannabinoids also have powerful anti-inflammatory and antioxidant actions that protect neurons from immune system attack.

According to several recent studies, endocannabinoids have many other functions in the brain and immune system. They include regulating development and aiding survival of young neurons, as well as controlling the wiring of neurons into circuits for learning and memory.

The intriguing research seems to suggest that people with a family history of Alzheimer's and who test positive for high-risk genes might consider talking to a doctor about using medical marijuana at moderate levels before symptoms arise.

But don't toke up. Despite these benefits, THC and other com-pounds in marijuana have many undesirable side effects on the brain, and smoking it in particular can be damaging. The weed itself is a complex witches' brew of many brain-altering chemicals. The cannabis plant contains about sixty different cannabinoids, so the challenge lies in trying to tease out which are the important ones for protecting neurons. The strength and composition of THC in plants also varies widely with how and where it's grown. The trick for scientists will be to isolate the active ingredients in marijuana that are beneficial and develop drugs that can be applied in the proper dose for the specific age of the patient. The beneficial effects of THC, for example, are in much lower concentrations of the chemical than are found in the plants people use to get high.

Several laboratories around the world are now investigating marijuana and Alzheimer's disease. In the meantime, Maria de Ceballos, a neurology researcher at the Cajal Institute in Madrid, is designing a study to see if those who indulge in the herb have lower rates of Alzheimer's disease. If so, the results might generate some serious buzz.

The Future—Without Alzheimer's Disease

Many of the research findings and the rate of medical progress on treating Alzheimer's disease are discouraging. But medical science has made amazing advances in lowering disease and death rates overall (remember the statistics on average longevity?). It has conquered many killers in the recent past. Consider: The federal government has invested in heart disease, HIV/AIDS, and certain cancers at an annual rate in the multiple billions of dollars. The death rates for these major killers are dropping due to positive, beneficial results in treatment.

Meanwhile, the death rate and financial burden from Alzheimer's skyrocket. Ironically, the sheer number of us reaching old old age may be part of the problem. As our brains, and worldwide population, age, the growing epidemic of Alzheimer's disease threatens to wreck the economy and health care systems. If dementia care were a country, it would be the world's eighteenth largest economy, ranking between Turkey and Indonesia. If it were a company, it would be the world's largest by annual revenue, exceeding Walmart ($414 billion) and Exxon Mobil ($311 billion), according to a 2010 report from Alzheimer's Disease International.

In the year 2010, the United States spent close to $172 billion for Alzheimer's care (70 percent through taxpayer-funded Medicare and Medicaid support) but $469 million for basic and translational research grants through the National Institutes of Health (NIH) that drive the search for the effective therapies that would reduce the costs of care. The 2012 proposed budget for Alzheimer's disease at the NIH is $458 million, which includes funding for basic research, clinical research, training, and support.

That puts the ratio of "cure" to "care" at about 1 to 400. These care costs will continue to escalate as a result of the aging demographics, with more than ten thousand people turning 65 every day for the next nineteen years, creating a larger at risk population.

Researchers and advocacy organizations say that counteracting Alzheimer's disease is going to take a much greater financial investment than current levels but that it will pay off both economically and socially.

Those of us in the danger years would certainly agree with that. We can contribute to the search for a cure by pushing for more research, participating in studies and trials, and perhaps donating our brains for study after death. (See the Resources section for more information.)

We might also begin by taking better care of our own aging brains.

PART THREE

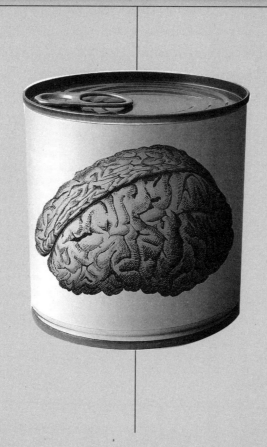

How to Optimize Your Aging Brain

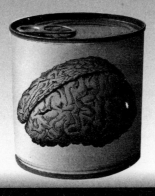

CHAPTER SIX

The Big Five for Optimal Brain Function

Can you keep a good brain from going bad? And help a faltering brain back to fighting trim?

It's possible. There's growing evidence that some lifestyle practices can slow or prevent issues that compromise your mental function and that changing some habits can help lower your risks of conditions that contribute to a battered brain. And it could be that some practices prevent or slow the progress of the most dreaded brain failing of old age, dementia.

Until recently, the evidence wasn't encouraging. In fact, when the National Institutes of Health (NIH) convened a panel of independent experts in August 2010 on how to prevent Alzheimer's disease, the conclusions were pretty grim. The panel determined that "no evidence of even moderate scientific quality" links anything—anything at all, from herbal or nutritional supplements to prescription medications to social, economic, environmental, or lifestyle conditions—with the slightest decrease in the risk of developing Alzheimer's disease. Furthermore, the committee agreed, little credible evidence exists that you can do anything to delay the kinds of memory problems often associated with aging.

The researchers' conclusions made headlines around the world and struck a blow at the many purveyors of "brain boosters," "memory enhancers," and "cognitive-training software" that advertise their wares on the Web and on television—part of a $291-billion-a-year industry. And they also struck fear in the hearts of many boomers and those who are older who have been counting on healthy lifestyle practices and brain training to ward off Alzheimer's and other brain issues of aging.

But did the panel overstate its case? Some memory and cognition researchers were critical, grumbling that the conclusions were too negative, particularly with respect to the potential benefits of not smoking, treating high blood pressure, and engaging in physical activity. All of these are known to reduce heart disease and a slew of other conditions that accompany or appear to contribute to dementia.

So they rejoiced when, less than a year after the NIH announcement, a contradictory report came out of the July 2011 Alzheimer's Association International Conference on Alzheimer's Disease in Paris.

Researchers from the University of California, San Francisco, used a mathematical model that predicted that up to half of the cases of Alzheimer's could be attributed to lifestyle choices and behaviors that could be modified. They are, in descending order of magnitude, lower education, smoking, physical inactivity, depression, midlife high blood pressure, diabetes, and midlife obesity.

The researchers were quick to point out that their conclusions are based on the assumption of a causal association between each risk factor and Alzheimer's and that such a connection hasn't been absolutely scientifically proven. Yet scientific evidence connects or associates each of these factors with increased risks of almost all of the conditions that contribute to dementia, and directly or indirectly to Alzheimer's disease itself.

It would be ideal if research today proved that exercise, good diet, and the other behaviors associated with a healthy body paid off to maintain a healthy elder brain. But ethics prevent getting better data through usual research methods. One of the best ways scientists have to prove cause and effect in medicine is to conduct a randomized controlled trial, in which study subjects are randomly assigned to two groups. The control group receives the usual standard of care; the experimental group gets whichever intervention is being tested. The simplest way, for example, to prove that treating high blood pressure helps to delay the onset of dementia would be to treat one group for hypertension and leave the other group with high blood pressure deliberately untreated for the sake of the experiment. No ethical physician would participate in such a study.

Moreover, pharmaceutical companies are not interested in funding studies on whether unpatentable substances, such as green tea or curcumin, or exercise might slow or halt the processes that lead to dementia.

We have been dependent on observational studies, which follow people as they get older—and that's where these associations show up. So while cause and effect isn't proven, there are strong associations between certain lifestyle factors that protect against dementia and with those that seem to accompany it.

The very good news is that these are, for the most part, issues you can do something about—right away, right now. Researchers are finding that you may lower the risks of developing dementia, delay the onset, or slow the progress even if it has begun. Getting regular exercise, staying socially engaged, participating in activities that make you think, and even having a positive attitude appear to have a meaningful influence on how effective your cognitive functioning will be in old age.

One major question for the lifestyle work is whether such interventions have different effects in people whose brains are currently normal than they do in those already showing Alzheimer's-related changes. They may help those who are healthy, but if you're already on the road—if you've got the genes, and you've already got a head full of amyloid—these interventions may be less able to slow the progression.

In coming years, rigorous government-funded clinical trials may show whether diet and exercise can delay the disease or whether the evidence from the epidemiology was just a statistical fluke. But if it turns out in some future research that these are not connected with dementia, you still will have improved your health overall, because all of these have vigorous scientific evidence that they can reduce disease in general, relieve many symptoms, ease stress and anxiety, lower heart disease, and make you feel and look all around better.

The Cognitive Shop

There's at least one formal program based on the lifestyle preventative approach. The families in Medellín, Colombia, with genetically based early-onset Alzheimer's have served as inspiration for an innovative approach to prevention in the United States: a "cognitive shop," known more formally as the center for Cognitive Fitness and Innovative Therapies (CFIT), in a residential neighborhood of Santa Barbara, California.

A refuge for both the worried well and those with mild memory complaints that sometimes precede full-fledged Alzheimer's, the center offers advice, based on the best existing evidence, about life changes and practices they can make that might perhaps help ward off the specter of dementia or help better cope with it if it does arrive.

Neuroscientist Kenneth S. Kosik, who has worked with the Colombian families for nearly twenty years, established the cognitive shop a few years ago, inspired by Casa Neurociencias, a less sumptuous outpatient clinic near the central hospital in Medellín. Patients with the genetic mutation for early-onset Alzheimer's, along with, at times, dozens of family members, would take a long bus ride from the countryside to spend the day in the clinic, where the medical staff and family members had easy access to one another. Kosik was impressed by the way the caring side and the ancillary services were available, even though the medical system was not so well developed.

Kosik contrasted the atmosphere favorably to the clinical efficiency of Harvard Medical School, where he had cofounded a memory disorders clinic at Brigham and Women's Hospital before moving to the University of California, Santa Barbara, in 2004. "I developed a frustration with the fact that people would come into the clinic and we would say, yes, this is looking like Alzheimer's, and then it was, adios," he says. "We would see them and follow up every six months, but we couldn't do much except document their decline."

CFIT in contrast offers lifestyle recommendations, much of them based on the still evolving body of scientific studies suggesting that nutrition, exercise, and other factors might help brain health. After a physical and psychological evaluation, a client (the word *patient* is never used) receives a series of personalized recommendations that may include adopting the Mediterranean diet (healthy fats and high fruit and vegetable consumption), engaging in aerobic exercise, and playing online brain games—activities that have yet to become standard practice at places such as the Harvard-affiliated memory clinic.

CFIT offers clients more control of their medical care. A cognitive psychologist guides people through the morass of medical information on the Internet, leading them through clinical trials or recent studies—on curcumin or other dietary supplements purported to protect brain cells, for example—explaining the weight of evidence.

And it offers the controversial practice of coordinating testing for the ApoE4 gene variant. The test is done after counseling the client about the implications of learning the results: if positive, not only they but also siblings and children may carry the same gene version and thus be at higher risk. Medical groups discourage testing because knowing gene status doesn't definitively predict about getting (or not) Alzheimer's and because there are no effective treatments.

To some scientists, these are startling and unorthodox practices. But Kosik, who was a coauthor of one of the early papers on the toxic tau protein, is hardly a physician who endorses flaky ideas. His laboratory at the University of California, Santa Barbara, does studies on the tau protein and other basic biology. At the very least, CFIT is intended to fill the gap until drugs or other measures have been proven to work.

"The solutions we have here are ultimately not the best solution," Kosik says. "But we don't know when a drug is going to arrive that

---

TAKING CARE OF MAINTENANCE:
SEE TO YOUR HEALTH ISSUES

A healthy brain needs a healthy body to move it around, and general overall health is connected with optimum brain function. So be sure at any age to see to the basics:

- Get a physical exam, and get tested yearly for blood pressure, cholesterol, glucose, and vitamin levels.
- Take care of your teeth. See a dentist at least twice a year.
- Keep up with inoculations for flu, pneumonia, and shingles.
- Know what medications you are taking and why, and ask your doctor yearly if they are necessary.
- Use protection during sex to avoid sexually transmitted diseases.
- Get enough good sleep: that's how the brain consolidates memories, and poor sleep is connected with cognitive issues.
- If you have a chronic condition, check in with your doctor regularly for what's new in treatments and to update your medication. Educate yourself: most conditions have associations and Web sites such as those for Alzheimer's disease, arthritis, diabetes, and heart disease.

treats the disease the same way penicillin treats an infection. I think it's irresponsible to tell people it's going to be five or ten years, because I don't think we know that."

How to Keep Your Brain Healthy and Nimble

While we don't know for certain what causes Alzheimer's and some other kinds of dementia or how to prevent memory loss and other cognitive failings, we do know that several unhealthy behaviors are connected with higher risks and rates of dementia—and that healthy activities are associated with healthy older brains.

For starters, what's good for the heart is good for the brain, a phrase that appears again and again in research. The same things that can cause arterial disease and heart attacks—high blood pressure, plaque buildup, arterial damage, atrial fibrillation—also contribute to strokes. So when you watch your cholesterol, control your blood pressure, maintain a healthy weight, and exercise for your heart, your brain benefits too. But research is also discovering tangible results from seeming intangibles such as attitude, intellectual exercise, and an active social life.

Here's what the experts say may help to preserve what you've got, minimize what you've lost, and lower the risks of Alzheimer's and other dementias.

Many agree that taking care of the five areas outlined here can help keep your brain and, incidentally, your body, at its personal best:

- *Physical activity:* Exercise daily for at least two and a half hours every week. This can be as simple as brisk walking. We'll do the math for you: that's about twenty-one minutes per day.
- *Mental stimulation:* Challenge your brain by learning something new and difficult. It needs to be hard for you, but it doesn't have to

be unpleasant. Learn a language, solve a puzzle, or teach a class, for example.

- *Nutrition:* Eat wisely, well—and less (obesity is connected with dementia). Dietary deficiencies sap your brain health.
- *Socialization:* People need people, and isolation and loneliness are connected with a weakened immune system and dementia.
- *Creativity, soul, and attitude:* Enrich thyself with artistic, religious, and spiritual practices, meditation, education, creativity, and an optimistic outlook—and lower stress.

Taking care of your overall health is also important. The Alzheimer Research Forum reports that three studies from separate groups in the July 2011 journal *Neurology* suggested that even minor ailments and illnesses associated with aging might hasten cognitive loss. The seemingly small issues "accumulate to turn into big risks," one researcher noted.

Among the conditions connected with cognitive decline were both high and low hemoglobin levels in older people that were tied to greater risk of Alzheimer's and faster rates of cognitive decline; high levels of proinflammatory cytokines, which contribute to systemic inflammation known to damage the brain; and the congregation of a number of issues not usually associated with dementia but connected with poor general health, such as poor eyesight, foot problems, nasal congestion, and wearing dentures.

These conditions and illnesses might be related to dementia because they are connected with other health behaviors, such as lack of physical activity and poor nutrition, the researchers speculate; or they may cause harm by stressing a brain already impaired. Whatever the reason, the evidence indicates it's important to take care of your overall health.

A word of caution: there's a lot of misinformation and downright false information out there about so-called alternative therapies, especially about supplements such as ginkgo biloba (found to be ineffective for supporting memory) and massive doses of vitamins (which can be dangerous to your health).

Some vitamin deficiencies can contribute to cognitive failings. But most supplements take your money and produce what more than one doctor has called "expensive urine." Be wary of inflated claims, and be sure to talk with your doctor before dosing yourself. (See "Is There a Pill for That?" in Chapter Nine.)

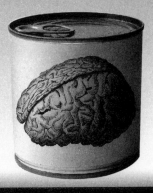

CHAPTER SEVEN

Exercise Your Body
Move Your Body for a Better Brain

Research has shown that your body loses muscle mass, strength, and health if you don't use it. Now we know that your brain also stays in better shape when you exercise your body—and that it's never too late to start.

Neuroscientists have known for a long time that physical exercise is related to brain health. In fact, exercise is a proven prescription for lowering the risks and the effects of many conditions that can hurt your brain, including high blood pressure and cholesterol, heart disease, stroke, type 2 diabetes, and depression. It also helps relieve stress, which has been shown to kill off brain cells (and is not so hot for the rest of your body either).

The newest research shows it may do even more. Aerobic exercise may halt or slow cognitive dysfunction, and provoke the growth of new brain cells in some areas and help your brain keep them. It makes your brain bigger, increasing volume in key areas that tend to shrink with age, including the gray and white matter volume in the prefrontal cortex and the hippocampus. And it increases the functioning of key nodes in your brain's executive control network.

So you might expect that daily physical exercise would maintain your brain by reducing risks of dementia, including Alzheimer's disease, and that's just what research in humans is beginning to show. Think of your brain as another muscle. Studies in animal models of aging have already shown that exercise can increase blood flow to the brain, stimulate nerve cell growth in regions associated with memory, and reduce the pathological changes characteristic of Alzheimer's disease, including, perhaps, memory loss. As a bonus, exercise stimulates the release of endorphins, the feel-good hormones.

THE MANY BRAIN BENEFITS OF EXERCISE

With so many powerful proven benefits, exercise should be a number one prescription. You knew this already, didn't you? But knowing is not doing, and disturbing research shows nearly 34 percent of Americans are obese and 25 percent inactive, conditions bad for that aging brain and aging heart.

Here's a reminder of what daily exercise can do for your brain health:

- Provoke production of new brain cells and increase brain volume in key areas
- Help reduce risks and effects of many conditions that contribute to dementia such as diabetes, stroke, and heart disease
- Help control weight and lower cholesterol and blood pressure
- Improve balance, which helps prevent falls, a major cause of brain injury in elders
- Lower stress, anxiety, and depression
- Promote good sleep, which is associated with good brain health

The positive impact of exercise adds to what we are learning about the heart-brain connection. While researchers know that physical exercise helps the brain, they haven't completely understood why on a biochemical level. One explanation, says Henrietta van Praag, a neurobiologist at the National Institute on Aging, is that exercising the heart somehow stimulates growth factors to produce new nerve cells in the brain. In 1999 van Praag, then at the Salk Institute in San Diego, showed that more new neurons formed in the hippocampus—one of the key centers in the brain for memory and learning—in physically active mice than in inactive ones. She has since shown that this new cell growth is associated with a marked improvement in learning and memory and that younger cells are better at establishing new connections with other cells.

The studies in humans are confirming this. Scientists are finding that older adults who participated in aerobic exercise such as walking outperformed those who were in programs for stretching and toning when both groups were tested for cognitive tasks in executive function (related to planning and multitasking), controlled responses to new situations, dealing with spatial information, and speed.

For instance, in a study published in 2001, neuropsychiatrist Kristine Yaffe of the University of California, San Francisco, and her colleagues recruited 5,925 women older than age 65 at four medical centers across the United States. The participants were all free of any physical disability that would limit their ability to walk or pursue other physical activities. They were also screened to ensure that they didn't have a cognitive impairment.

The researchers then assessed the physical activity of these women by asking them how many city blocks they walked and how many flights of stairs they climbed daily and gave them a questionnaire to fill out about their levels of participation in thirty-three physical activities. Six to eight years later, the researchers assessed the women's level of cognitive function. The women who reported the most activity had a 30 percent lower risk of cognitive decline. Interestingly, walking distance, but not walking speed, was related to cognition. It seemed that even moderate levels of physical activity may serve to limit declines in cognition in these older adults.

This Brain Was Made for Walking

Could it be that simple—that a walk a day can keep Alzheimer's disease away? Several studies suggest it could be so. In fact, a recent study shows that just plain walking, and not even that much of it, can make your brain not just better but also bigger, especially in the areas devoted to memory making. For those who are intimidated by a gym (not to mention its costs), here's a therapy that's free, available anywhere and at any time, and now proven to improve your memory and perhaps delay dementia.

Researchers know that the volume of both the hippocampus and medial temporal lobe shrink with age, beginning in late adulthood, and that this is associated with impaired memory and increased risks for dementia. They also know that these areas are larger in more fit adults, but didn't know if—or how much—exercise could help in later adult years.

Quite a bit, it seems. A 2010 controlled trial based on walking a mere two hours a week revealed that at least some parts of the brain can be saved from atrophy—and even built up—by relatively modest amounts of activity in later years.

A research team recruited 120 previously sedentary adults aged 55 to 80 years who didn't have diagnosable dementia but did show typical age-related shrinking of the hippocampus according to prestudy magnetic resonance imaging (MRI). They were put into two groups: one group walked around a track for forty minutes three days a week and the other group did stretching exercises.

At the end of a year, MRIs showed that the walking group increased the volume of the hippocampus by 2.12 percent in the left hippocampus and 1.97 percent in the right hippocampus—a modest increase, but one that researchers say effectively turned back the clock one to two years in terms of brain volume. The older adults assigned to a stretching routine showed no such growth. In fact, they lost volume: on average 1.40 percent and 1.43 percent in the volume of their left and right hippocampus, respectively.

And although both groups improved in accuracy on memory tests, the walking group did better on memory tests, which also correlated with the hippocampus growth. Those who were in better shape (and thus tended to have a larger hippocampus) at the start of the study did the best on the later memory tests. The walking group also tended to have a higher level of brain-derived neurotrophic factor (BDNF), a compound associated with having a larger hippocampus and better memory.

The researchers didn't see any changes in the thalamus or caudate nucleus, two other parts of the brain involved with spatial sense and memory, respectively. Because only the hippocampus seemed to be affected by the walking regime, the researchers reasoned that the activity might be acting specifically on certain molecular pathways to prompt cell proliferation or dendritic branching.

It's Never Too Late to Start Exercising

Discoveries about the brain's impressive ability to change and compensate for damaged areas are being reported almost daily. Even so, the new findings on the value of exercise are astounding. They show that even at a relatively advanced age—perhaps your age—the brain remains remarkably plastic in key structural areas.

The walking studies, for example, tell us that it's never too late. Although being in better shape to begin with is linked to better memory, starting an exercise regimen later in life can pay off in brain benefits even when some cognitive decline has already set in.

Researchers at the University of Pittsburgh found that walking five to six miles a day slows the progress of dementia in those who are already showing mild cognitive impairment (MCI) or Alzheimer's disease. The participants in an ongoing twenty-year study were recruited from a Cardiovascular Heart Study, where they were monitored for how much and far they walked weekly. Of the 426 adults, 299 (mean age of 78) were healthy, 127 (mean age of 81) had some

---

WHAT KIND OF EXERCISE?

Experts say we need a minimum of two and half hours a week or thirty minutes a day of brisk exercise. The kind of exercise depends on you, and there are plenty of choices. Just about anything that gets you moving, preferably moving hard enough to work up a light sweat and raise your heart rate, is good for you, including walking. Some studies show benefits from pumping up your heart rate and respiration, but others suggest it's not the intensity but the regularity and length of the workout.

That gives plenty of latitude. Let us list some of the ways:

- *Activities of daily living* can meet some of your workout requirements, especially if you live in a three-story home and trek up and down the stairs several times a day. Other ordinary activities include mowing the lawn with a push mower, gardening, and vigorous cleaning. But these alone are probably not enough.

- *Walking, walking, walking.* We have to repeat it: a clutch of new studies says about five miles a week or so is associated with lower risks of dementia, along with the other known benefits.

- *Get wet.* Swimming and aquatic aerobics work your joints and your muscles without the drag of gravity. If you have arthritis or other painful conditions, look for a warm-water pool near you. Canoeing and kayaking are terrific any-age sports.

cognitive impairment, and 123 already had either MCI or Alzheimer's disease.

Researchers used brain scans and mental tests to note changes. The findings: those with the greater amount of exercise had the greater brain volume and better scores on mental exams, and that included those who already had cognitive issues. In fact, those who already had cognitive decline and exercised lost only an average of one point on the tests, whereas those who were not as active declined by five points.

- *Biking.* A ride with the grandkids or your friends is great (protect your brain with a helmet). If you have uncertain balance, try a stationary bike, at a high resistance, for five or more miles (twenty minutes) daily.

- *Court sports.* Those whose knees are up to it revel in tennis, volleyball, handball, racket ball, and badminton. The eye-hand coordination required is a plus.

- *Dance or aerobics* classes exercise your brain as well, especially partnered dances such as the tango. Tap and ballet are good at any age, and so is jazzercise.

- *Cross-country skiing* uses thousands of calories and most of your muscle groups, and it is safer than downhill skiing.

- *Tai chi,* the ancient Chinese program of smoothly choreographed movements, can be done at any age and has been shown to improve balance, lower blood glucose levels and blood pressure, and improve immune function.

- *Yoga* increases flexibility and strength, reduces blood pressure, and the other health benefits of this ancient practice are well documented. It pairs nicely with cardiovascular activities that raise your heart rate, and with meditation, which lowers stress. In fact, both yoga and tai chi have been called "moving meditations."

A 2008 a study from the University of Western Australia showed similar improvements in those who already have memory issues. They studied 170 older people with memory complaints, including 60 diagnosed with MCI. Half the group was encouraged to do at least three fifty-minute sessions of exercise (mostly walking) each week. (Those already doing this level of exercise added fifty minutes to their existing regime.) The other half got basic health education as a control group.

At the end of six months, exercisers improved modestly (scoring about 20 percent higher than controls), including the subgroup with MCI. A year after the trial ended, the exercisers still sustained a 10 percent edge on overall cognitive scores and had significantly less memory decline.

Walking also helps if you already have vascular disease, high blood pressure, and other heart issues known to contribute to cognitive decline. In yet another study, 2,809 women age 65 or older with vascular disease or at least three coronary risk factors were studied over almost five and a half years. The study interviewed women by phone about their physical activity and tested them for memory and other cognitive changes three times over the years, comparing the scores with physical activity. They found that those who said they exercised the equivalent of walking briskly for at least thirty minutes every day significantly slowed mental losses—and those who reported the highest levels of exercising tested the equivalent of being mentally five to seven years younger.

Here's more proof that it's never too late. In 2003 psychiatrist Marcus Richards of University College London and his colleagues studied the influence of self-reported physical exercise and leisure-time activities on memory in 1,919 men and women at two ages: they looked at memory changes between ages 36 and 43 and at changes from ages 43 to 53. And, lo, physical exercise and other leisure-time activities at age 36 were associated with higher memory scores at age

43, and a slower rate of memory decline from ages 43 to 53 (after adjusting for variables).

And here's a show-stopper: the data also suggest there's little memory protection for those who stopped exercising after age 36 but protection for those who *began* to exercise after then. In 2005, Suvi Rovio, then a graduate student at the Karolinska Institute in Sweden, and her colleagues examined the relation between physical activity at middle age and risk of dementia an average of twenty-one years later, when the cohort was between 65 and 79 years of age. Subjects indicated how often they participated in leisure-time physical activities that lasted at least twenty to thirty minutes and caused breathlessness and sweating. Activity at least twice a week at midlife was associated with a reduced risk of dementia in later life. Indeed, those in the more active group had 52 percent lower odds of having dementia than the more sedentary group did.

How about after age 70? A study that examined the relation between physical activity and cognitive change over a two-year period in 16,466 nurses older than 70 years found a significant relation between the amount of energy expended in physical activities and in cognitive abilities.

A Fine Balance: Yoga, Tai Chi, and Fall Prevention

Falling—even a simple, ordinary tumble that bangs the head—is the most common cause of serious brain injury in seniors. Such brain damage accounts for 46 percent of the fatalities from falls among older adults. One out of every three people over age 65 takes a fall each year, and about 60 percent of older adults with cognitive impairment suffer at least one fall each year.

The Centers for Disease Control considers it such a problem that it has an entire program on how to prevent seniors from falling. And at the top of the list is a regular exercise program to build strength and improve balance and coordination. Yoga and tai chi are darn near perfect for that.

For thousands of years, people in Asia have practiced both for healthy mind and body, and research has backed up their value. Practiced gently, they ease the frail and sedentary into movement and flexibility. Practiced on an expert level, these can be effective aerobic exercises. Practiced on any level, they contribute to mobility, balance, and mood.

Yoga has become wildly popular in the West, and tai chi, practiced daily by hundreds of millions worldwide and daily in parks throughout China, has also been embraced by Westerners and been proven to help with mobility and balance issues. In recent years, studies have found both yoga and tai chi to lower stress and blood pressure, improve depression and anxiety, and lower inflammation, all issues that contribute to dementia. Tai chi is even connected to lowering the blood glucose level for those with diabetes, and yoga has been shown to improve balance after stroke. And here's a plus: the concentration involved to master the routines also exercises the brain, can yield some of the benefits of meditation, and improves memory. These are best when paired with regular cardio exercise that raises your heart rate, such as walking briskly or biking.

Don't try to learn these from a book or video. These are great for experienced practitioners, but for beginners, it's best to first attend classes to learn correct and safe alignment and technique. There's such a range of athleticism in both of these practices that it's wise to choose your classes and your instructors carefully, based on your level of fitness. Classes at your gym or health club may be too demanding and vigorous (although most are not). Your health maintenance organization or local health center probably offers classes in both, or check with your doctor or a local senior center.

The Yale Program in Geriatrics also recommends reducing medications (if possible) and avoiding alcohol, since both can affect balance, and increasing vitamin D (for bone health).

FEAR OF FALLING CRIPPLES

Broken spirits, not bones, may be the worst result of falling. Many older people fall, and for some, the experience makes them so afraid of toppling again that their mind impairs their ability to walk without trembling or losing balance. They quickly make themselves dependent on canes or wheelchairs.

Roger Kurlan, a neurologist at the University of Rochester, has seen about thirty cases of what he calls "fear-of-falling gait." The condition may also make individuals vulnerable to dangerous misdiagnoses. The doctor of one 76-year-old woman noticed her tremor and inability to walk unaided and prescribed medication—wrongly—for Parkinson's disease. But after talking with her, Kurlan managed to get her out of her wheelchair, and she was soon walking securely around his office. He is now encouraging physicians who spot such symptoms to ask patients about recent falls instead of assuming a neurological problem and prescribing unnecessary medication, physical therapy, or even institutionalization.

Another recipe for improved balance, and the enjoyment of exercise, is to add music and stir things up. Scientists in Switzerland recruited 134 adults with an average age of about 75, almost all of them women. For six months, half took a weekly hour-long class that focused on balance, working out to piano music, and changing movements in response to changes in the beat. The exercises became progressively more difficult. Meanwhile, the other group continued with their regular activities for six months.

Those who worked out to tunes improved their gait and had longer and more stable strides, according to Andrea Trombetti and colleagues. Then the two groups switched. Overall, the first music-exercising group experienced half as many falls as the control group. But when the control group started striding to songs six months in, they gained the same benefits: improved gait and longer and more stable strides.

Madeleine E. Hackney and Gammon M. Earhart of the Washington University School of Medicine have also shown you can dance your way to better balance. Their studies with partnered tango and fox-trot dancing sessions found dance improved balance and gait in people with mild to moderate Parkinson's disease.

A bonus is that all of these activities are social and enjoyable—more good news for your brain.

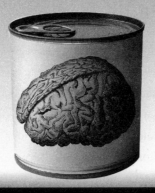

CHAPTER EIGHT

Challenge Your Brain

Neurologists have been producing studies for decades that suggest that adults who regularly challenge their brains stay sharper: they succumb to dementia less often, less severely, and at older ages than seniors who are—how do we say this?—intellectually lazy. They've also learned that the mature brain is still plastic, even one with mild cognitive impairment. If it gets a workout, it can grow new neural connections and strengthen weak ones.

"Workout" is the key: the brain must be challenged. It has to work at something new and very hard. Repeating something you already know, even if it is difficult, may not stretch your brain enough. John Adams, one of the longest-lived U.S. presidents, who died at age 91, put it this way: "Old minds are like old horses; you must exercise them if you wish to keep them in working order."

How best to keep minds keen over an entire life span is a question philosophers have mulled over since the earliest writings on record, and one that scientists are pursuing with zeal in today's aging population. Remember: their brains are aging, too. Back in the 1970s and 1980s, research showed that healthy older adults could improve their mental as well as physical performance more than had ever before been believed. But only in recent years has research begun showing that specific cognitive training could substantially benefit older brains, that these effects can be relatively long lasting, and that those studies can apply to most of us. It seems that newly learned skills can be developed in specific areas, can be retained, and can influence the thinking skills needed in everyday life.

Around the turn of this century, the federal government's National Institute on Aging funded a consortium of researchers to conduct a large-scale training study in a sample of older Americans. In 2002 psychologist Karlene Ball of the University of Alabama at Birmingham and her colleagues published initial results on a study of twenty-five hundred people older than age 65 who had received about ten sessions of cognitive training. They had been randomly assigned to a cognitive-process training group to learn how to excel in one of three areas—memory, reasoning, or visual search—or to a control group that didn't get training.

At follow-ups two years and five years later, the team randomly selected a group to get booster training before being evaluated. They found strong performance improvements in the experimental group—but only in the specific areas of training, a typical finding in research on brain training. For example, those trained in visual search had strong gains in visual search performance but little improvement, compared to the control group, on the memory and reasoning tests.

More impressive are recent training exercises that focus on executive function—the thinking skills used in planning a strategic approach to a task and how we manage the mind in the process. Unlike the training that focused on very specific skills, such as memorization strategies, the exercises that aim to help people control how they think appears to work on broader skills that are helpful in many situations.

For instance, psychologist Chandramallika Basak and her colleagues at the University of Illinois recently showed that training with a real-time strategy video game that demands planning and executive control improved not only game performance but performance on other executive control tasks.

You don't have to have specialized brain exercises, however, to achieve cognitive gains that may help ward off cognitive decline. More than a dozen studies suggest that even everyday activities such as reading can help. In 2003 neuropsychologist Robert S. Wilson and his colleagues at Rush University Medical Center in Chicago recruited more than four thousand elders from a geographically defined community and rated how often they participated in seven cognitive activities—for instance, reading magazines. At three-year intervals for nearly six years, the participants completed an in-home interview that included brief tests of cognitive function. And, of course, the more frequently they were involved in cognitive activity at the outset, the lower the rate was of cognitive decline.

The rule seems to be: learn something new and hard. This may not always be fun. In his book, *Healthy Aging,* wellness guru and doctor Andrew Weil recommends learning a new computer operating system or skill (or using a computer if you don't already) or another language. If that makes you groan out loud, remember: no pain, no gain. As Weil, who was born in 1942, says, the effort involved shows your brain is working hard.

Educated Brains Stay Better Longer

Regardless of brain-training exercises, studies also show that the more educated your brain is, the better it fares in later life. It wards off dementia longer, perhaps even after the brain has been riddled with beta-amyloid and other symptoms of Alzheimer's disease.

Catherine M. Roe and colleagues at Washington University studied nearly two hundred seniors (mean age 67) over a five-year period; thirty-seven of them had been diagnosed with Alzheimer's disease. They were injected with a radioactive substance, Pittsburgh compound B, which shows brain damage in imaging scans because it attaches to deposits of beta-amyloid, the toxic protein that forms plaques in the brains of those with the disease.

Some of the brains absorbed a lot of Pittsburgh compound B, an indication that these were riddled with beta-amyloid plaques. But regardless of these results, the more years of education participants had, the less likely they were to perform poorly on memory and thinking tests. In other words, their education seemed to protect them against the memory loss and other symptoms of Alzheimer's disease despite the presence of plaques.

If that education included another language, *tres bien*! Knowing two languages is better than knowing only one when it comes to warding off or delaying Alzheimer's, it seems. Ellen Bialystok and colleagues conducted two studies comparing healthy bilingual to monolingual brains. The first showed that older adults who spoke two languages performed better on tests of executive control. The second study examined the medical records of about four hundred people who already had Alzheimer's and *voilà:* the bilingual brains showed Alzheimer's symptoms five to fix years later than those who spoke one language.

Why Testing Boosts Learning

Researchers are confirming something we learned in grade school: that taking tests boosts learning. For more than a century, scientists have known that when we're tested on material, we're more likely to remember it than material we simply study.

Kent State University psychology researcher Katherine Rawson says that part of the explanation is that testing gets people to come up with better keyword clues. These clues bridge the gap between familiar and new information and strengthen ties between these keywords and the newly learned information.

Rawson and former graduate student Mary Pyc asked 118 college students to learn four dozen Swahili words by matching them with their English counterparts, such as *wingu,* which means "cloud." After an initial study period, half were given practice tests before studying the words a second time, and half restudied the words without taking a practice test. As expected, students in the practice test group were better at remembering the word pairs during a final exam a week later.

Rawson and Pyc also asked students to tell them their keywords—for instance, *bird* might serve as a bridge between *wingu* and *cloud.* They discovered that the people in the practice test group not only remembered more of their keywords but were more likely to have changed their keyword before restudying the word pairs than those who had not been tested. So testing may be just the ticket to better memory.

Do Brain Fitness Products Work?

Computerized brain-training games seem like a cool idea. The hype goes like this: build up you brain while you play and practice at home, usually on a computer, and ward off dementia and memory loss. The sales pitch for most of these programs is based in large part on evidence that living in an enriched environment with lots of mental stimulation produces positive brain changes. But do these sometimes-pricey products provide that kind of stimulation—and are they worth the money and the effort?

Cognitive training is growing in popularity as baby boomers age, and it's a boon for business as well. From 2005 to 2008, the U.S. brain fitness business increased from $100 million to $265 million and is expected to skyrocket, with revenue projected to leap to between $1 and $5 billion by 2015, according to a report by Marketwatch based on data from SharpBrains, a San Francisco company that tracks the cognitive-fitness industry. Even some insurers are getting in on the trend.

This extraordinary growth was driven at first by the early success of Nintendo's "Brain Age" and other brain-training games. Research does confirm that regular brain exercise—in the laboratory at least—is beneficial to elderly people. ACTIVE (Advanced Cognitive Training for Independent and Vital Elderly), a nationwide clinical trial of 2,802 seniors that began in 1998, found that training in specific areas such as processing speed resulted in improvements that persisted at least five years.

But while studies show promising results from such laboratory exercises, the commercial products are (so far) a different story. Reviewers for *Scientific American* have found that actual scientific evidence for most of them is scanty.

There have been few studies and mixed reports about their effectiveness. Even as the market for brain-training software continues to grow, evidence remains scarce as to the programs' ability to boost memory or intelligence in a broadly applicable way rather than simply making users better at the task they're practicing. New studies offer a tantalizing suggestion that certain programs may work, but the bulk of the research is murky.

In 2009, neuroscientist Peter Snyder of Brown University reviewed nearly twenty software studies and concluded that as a group, they were underwhelming. He found them marred by flaws such as a lack of control groups and follow-up. More than a third of those he reviewed were too shoddy even to include in the analysis he submitted that year in the journal *Alzheimer's and Dementia*. Although some products claimed to treat dementia, Snyder didn't find any evidence to back such claims.

One study did exceed expectations. In a study Snyder called the "most well-designed" of those he evaluated in 2009, the Mayo Clinic tested the Brain Fitness Program by Posit Science. "This is a good first study to emerge out of a terribly messy literature," he said, and he'd like to see if it can be replicated. Encouragingly, the researchers found that the software boosted the brain in ways unrelated to the training. Rather than simply learning to parrot back what they had practiced, participants improved their test scores across a range of brain functions. People who used the program bolstered their working memory—the system that holds information in mind momentarily in tasks such as dialing phone numbers—and processing speed, two assets that deteriorate with age.

Still, the boost was minimal. Players improved their memory by twice as much as the control group, but after eight weeks of training, that improvement was only about 4 percent.

Small effects such as those are a hallmark of brain-training software studies, Snyder says. But even though the improvement may be small, the effect on the brain is visible, according to a 2009 study. Neuroscientists at the Karolinska Institute in Sweden used positron emission tomography and functional magnetic resonance imaging scans to reveal changes in the number of receptors for dopamine—a chemical messenger involved in learning, among other important functions. Whether volunteers started with a relatively low or relatively high number of dopamine receptors, brain training resulted in a shift closer to the optimum balance.

Snyder praised Klingberg's study but also pointed out that it is a given that the brain will change in response to a variety of interventions. From his perspective, software companies remain hard-pressed to prove their products do much, especially over the long term, and few programs have demonstrated the flexibility to boost skills that were not practiced. "The evidence isn't in," Snyder cautions.

HOW TO GIVE YOUR BRAIN A WORKOUT

The more educated you are, the later you develop Alzheimer's disease, it seems. And the more mentally active you stay, the longer you stay mentally active. The anti-aging industry has figured this out and is selling a multimillion-dollar range of programs touted to improve your brain.

But you don't need pricey brain programs to give your noggin a workout. There's plenty you can do—but be sure it's hard for your individual brain. If you are an ace at the daily crossword puzzle, for example, that is not going to stretch your brain very much. Problem solving will use your mental networks, as will activities that force you to think in a different way.

Consider these:

- Study a language. Study shows bilingual people are at lower risk for Alzheimer's disease.

- Play chess, bridge, and other games that call on memory and reason.

- Get a computer (if you haven't already) and get online, where you will find free-of-charge brain games.

- Take up a musical instrument.

- Take a class. Better yet, teach a class. That really gets you on your mental toes.

Scientific American writer Kaspar Mossman, who tried a clutch of brain programs for eight weeks in 2009, concluded he learned some useful things about the software but didn't feel any smarter. That may be because he is still on the south side of aging and doesn't have any cognitive issues. If you have a serious problem, say some executives in the brain game business, the training is worth a lot more.

Perhaps. We already know the brain will change in response to a variety of interventions, and these are everywhere around us. So software companies remain hard-pressed to prove their products do much more, especially over the long term.

Computer Training May Keep You Driving Longer

Giving up the keys is a threshold moment for most seniors and can be start of a downward spiral. It's admitting your brain and its accessories, hearing and vision, aren't good enough anymore. And it can mean giving up a big chunk of independence.

But when is it time? Those of us on the far side of 50 may have noticed it already: our vision behind the wheel isn't what it used to be. That may be especially true for what's called the useful field of view (UFOV), the visual area you can see without moving your eyes or head. Diminished UFOVs have been correlated with a higher probability of getting into an accident.

Some age-related decline in visual performance is irreversible, but that doesn't mean there's nothing to be done about it. The right type of exercise may beef up neurons and connections, thicken myelin sheaths, and speed up performance in the brain's visual cortex, leading to better vision and quicker reaction time.

This is where some computer-training programs might come in. Clinical trials such as ACTIVE have shown that regular use of these programs can improve general cognitive function. Something similar can happen with visual processing as well.

In a 2003 paper in the journal *Nature,* psychologist Shawn Green and neuroscientist Daphne Bavelier of the University of Rochester found that playing commercial action video games such as Medal of Honor improved markers of visual processing, including UFOV. According to Green and Bavelier, playing such games "is capable of radically altering visual attentional processing." But while intense action and driving games like Grand Theft Auto can improve skills such as object-based attention, they're probably a bit too fast-paced and gory (not to mention rather unpleasant) for most older drivers.

When you drive, more than just one brain region is involved. Your eyes send information to the primary visual cortex and other parts of the occipital lobe. Processed data then move to the parietal lobe, which deals with orientation and attention. The frontal lobes make decisions and command the motor cortex to hit the brake if a pedestrian is in front of the car.

The problem, according to clinical neuroscientist Peter Snyder, is that measuring improvements in specific tasks is difficult, because the tests to do so are too similar to the tasks themselves. But with visual processing (as opposed to cognition), Snyder says, it is likely that we will be able to get a straight answer, because the training is so different from actual driving.

Some companies that provide cognitive-training software also offer products for people who specifically want to improve their visual system. As for whether these programs help to improve driving, Snyder says that "it's a hell of a lot easier to measure progress in a driving simulator than to design studies to determine whether older people think better." He is "guardedly optimistic" that some senior-driving programs might work as their makers claim.

At least one insurance company, Allstate, has partnered with a program from Posit Science in an ongoing study to see if its InSight program helps drivers over the age of 50. More than five thousand Allstate customers in Pennsylvania trained with InSight. The company is currently comparing the accident numbers of these drivers with those of a control group. "If completing the software does indeed improve driving," says Krissy Posey, an Allstate spokesperson, "Allstate hopes to offer discounts to drivers."

However, the training offer may not be wholly benevolent: the flip side could be that premiums would rise for those who fail the UFOV test or can't complete the program.

The Bottom Line

Before you invest your time and money, consider this: none of these programs may be as good as exercising your brain on your own— by playing chess, say, or learning to play a musical instrument or by

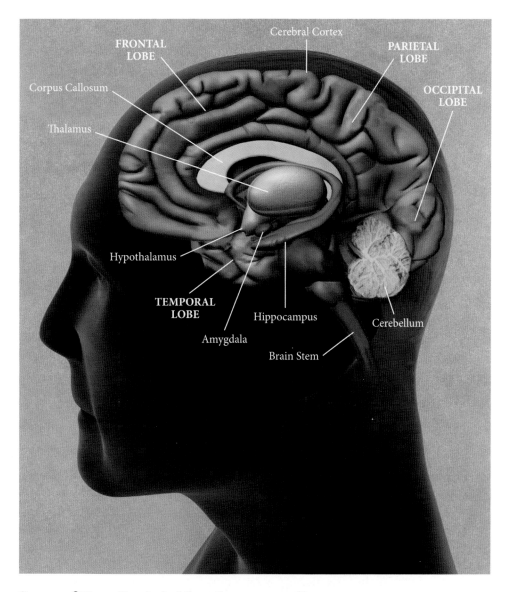

Some of Your Brain's Most Important Parts

Of course, all parts of your brain are important. Some appear more vulnerable to the effects of normal aging and dementia: the hippocampus, which is the gateway for learning and memory, and the cerebral cortex, the outermost part of the brain, which is responsible for thinking and making decisions.

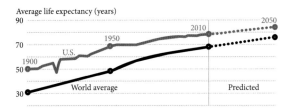

Average life expectancy (years)

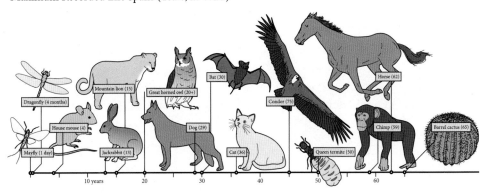

Maximum Recorded Life Spans (Years, in Wild)

Why Can't We Live Forever?

Throughout history, we know some people have lived to 100 years or more, but they were the exception. Today, centenarians are the fastest-growing age group, thanks largely to advances in medicine and sanitation that have extended life spans just about everywhere around the world. (See chart.) In the United States it has nearly doubled: around the beginning of the last century, the average person lived to be around 47; today the global average is 68—and in the United States it is into the 80s. For a 65-year-old woman it's around 85.

As the average life span of humans continues to lengthen, some scientists have begun to ponder whether this trend will continue indefinitely. After all, some species live two hundred years or more, and some research suggests that drugs or changes in diet may slow metabolism or alter basic aging processes so that we can live longer.

Evidence suggests, however, that biological constraints keep most species from surpassing age limits specific to that species: see the chart for some of the maximum recorded life spans of humans and of other animals in the wild.

It appears that the maximum age for a species depends on both biology (simpler organisms can reach Methuselean ages that more complex creatures cannot) and environment (dangerous surroundings lead to evolution of rapid reproduction, fast aging, and early death). The theories propose that life span is affected by the number of times cells can divide, and that number is limited.

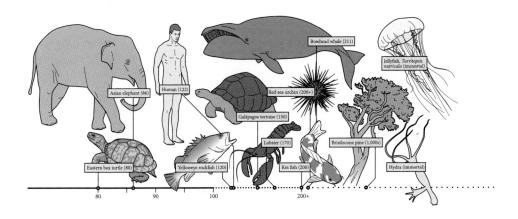

Asian elephant (86)

Human (122)

Bowhead whale (211)

Jellyfish, *Turritopsis nutricula* (immortal)

Red sea urchin (200+)

Galápagos tortoise (150)

Eastern box turtle (80)

Yelloweye rockfish (120)

Lobster (170)

Koi fish (200)

Bristlecone pine (1,000s)

Hydra (immortal)

80   90   100   200+

No one yet knows how to slow human aging, and all proposed longevity strategies remain unproved. Calorie restriction lengthens the life span of flies, worms, and mice over that of animals eating a normal diet. It's unclear yet whether caloric restriction can work in humans—or whether we'd enjoy life on ultra low calorie diets.

Basic research might eventually yield longevity drugs. Some compounds might tinker with cell metabolism (energy use) to mimic benefits seen in animals; others might change the way damaged cells behave. Investigators hope such interventions will extend today's maximum achievable life span—or at least help people stay healthy longer than they do now.

How the Brain Makes New Neurons

New cells in the brain are made from neural stem cells that divide periodically in two main areas: the ventricles (purple, inset), which contain cerebrospinal fluid to nourish the central nervous system, and the hippocampus (light blue, inset), crucial for learning and memory. The neural stem cells proliferate (cell pathways below) and give rise to other neural stem cells and to neural precursors that can grow up to be either neurons or glial cells. But these newborn neural stem cells need to move (red arrows, inset) away from their parents before they can differentiate. Only 50 percent, on average, survive; the others perish. In an adult brain, newborn neurons have been found in the hippocampus and the olfactory bulbs, which process smell.

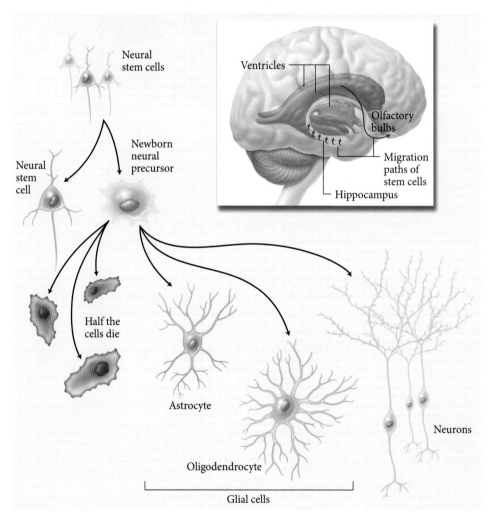

Neural stem cells

Ventricles

Olfactory bulbs

Newborn neural precursor

Neural stem cell

Migration paths of stem cells

Hippocampus

Half the cells die

Astrocyte

Neurons

Oligodendrocyte

Glial cells

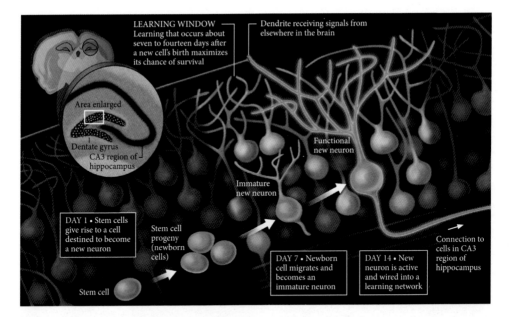

LEARNING WINDOW
Learning that occurs about seven to fourteen days after a new cell's birth maximizes its chance of survival

Dendrite receiving signals from elsewhere in the brain

Area enlarged

Dentate gyrus
CA3 region of hippocampus

Functional new neuron

Immature new neuron

DAY 1 • Stem cells give rise to a cell destined to become a new neuron

Stem cell progeny (newborn cells)

DAY 7 • Newborn cell migrates and becomes an immature neuron

DAY 14 • New neuron is active and wired into a learning network

Connection to cells in CA3 region of hippocampus

Stem cell

How Learning Helps Save New Neurons

During their first weeks of life, newborn brain cells in the hippocampus migrate from the edge of the dentate gyrus (where they are born) into a deeper area, where they mature and become wired into a network of neurons. Research shows that learning when the cells are about one to two weeks old enhances their survival. If there is no learning activity, most new hippocampus neurons die. Researchers hope to be able to induce an adult brain to repair itself by coaxing neural stem cells or neural precursors to divide and develop when and where they are needed.

How Myelin Is Made

Your brain talks to itself and collects information by sending messages between neurons on long arms called axons. When those axons are wrapped and insulated with myelin, the signals race to their targets much faster than on unmyelinated axons. Without myelin, the signal leaks and dissipates.

Glial cells in the white matter called oligodendrocyte cells manufacture the fatty insulating membrane and wrap the axons with 10 to 150 layers. Glial cells called astrocytes sometimes "listen in" on the signals traveling along axons and relay chemical messages to the oligodendrocytes.

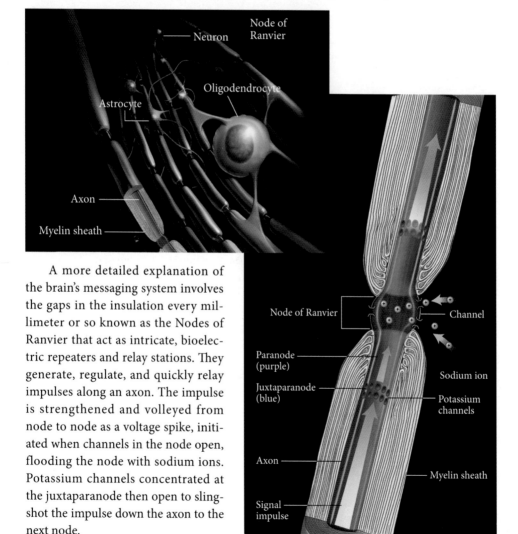

Neuron

Node of Ranvier

Oligodendrocyte

Astrocyte

Axon

Myelin sheath

Node of Ranvier

Channel

Paranode (purple)

Juxtaparanode (blue)

Sodium ion

Potassium channels

Axon

Myelin sheath

Signal impulse

A more detailed explanation of the brain's messaging system involves the gaps in the insulation every millimeter or so known as the Nodes of Ranvier that act as intricate, bioelectric repeaters and relay stations. They generate, regulate, and quickly relay impulses along an axon. The impulse is strengthened and volleyed from node to node as a voltage spike, initiated when channels in the node open, flooding the node with sodium ions. Potassium channels concentrated at the juxtaparanode then open to slingshot the impulse down the axon to the next node.

Glial Cells and Neurons: A Working Partnership

Your brain is made up just about 50–50 with white matter (glial cells) and gray matter (neurons). Although gray matter controls the brain's thinking and calculating, white matter controls the signals that neurons share, coordinating how well brain regions work together. Glia and neurons work together to speed information through the brain and spinal cord. A neuron (brain cell) sends an outgoing message down a long axon and across a synaptic gap to a receiving dendrite on another neuron. Several types of glial cells help with transmission. Astrocyte glia bring nutrients to neurons as well as surround and regulate synapses. Oligodendrocyte glia produce myelin that insulates axons. In the body's peripheral nervous system, Schwann cells perform myelination duties.

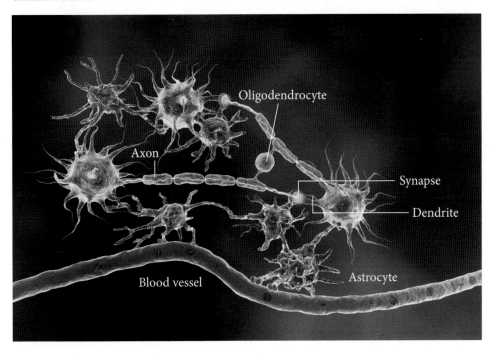

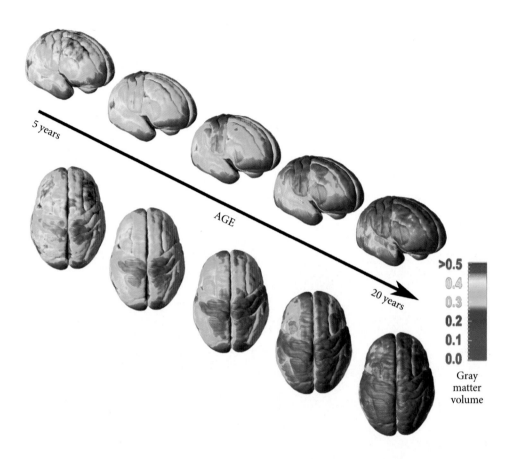

5 years

AGE

20 years

>0.5
0.4
0.3
0.2
0.1
0.0

Gray
matter
volume

Less Is More in Brain Development

The human brain is a work in process, not maturing until we are in our early 20s. As it grows, the balance between gray matter and white matter shifts: excess neurons are pruned away and myelin gradually increases, until they are roughly 50–50.

That balance is vital to a functioning brain. Cognitive function—thinking—depends on communication among neurons across synapses in the cortex's gray matter; and optimal communication among brain regions, which is also fundamental to proper cognition, depends on the white matter bedrock connecting the regions.

Myelin is only partially formed at birth and gradually develops in different regions, expands in spurts, and is not fully laid until age 25 or 30 in certain places. The timing of growth and degree of completion can affect learning, self-control (and why teenagers may lack it), and mental illnesses such as schizophrenia, autism, and even pathological lying.

Myelination generally proceeds in a wave from the back of the cerebral cortex (shirt collar) to its front (forehead) as we grow into adulthood, with the frontal lobes last. These regions are responsible for higher-level reasoning, planning, and judgment—skills that come only with experience. Once axons are myelinated, the changes they can undergo become more limited.

To trace the development of the human brain, researchers at the National Institute of Mental Health recruited thirteen children to undergo magnetic resonance imaging (MRI) brain scans every two years for eight to ten years to produce a time-lapse sequence of brain development.

The sequence here, by Paul Thompson of the University of California, Los Angeles, depicts the pruning of neurons and the relative increase in myelin in two views—right lateral and top—of how gray matter matures over the cortical surface from the age of 5 to 20. The color bar on the right represents the volume of gray matter in units. The imaging study reveals progressive "thinning" of gray matter in a wave that starts at the back of the brain and progresses to the front. Those regions that mature last—not until early adulthood—are associated with higher-order functions such as planning, reasoning, and impulse control.

Stroke: The Brain Attack

Stroke is the number-one cause of disability and a contributor to dementia. It does its damage by interrupting blood flow and starving the brain of oxygen, killing neurons.

There are two kinds of stroke. An ischemic stroke, shown here, is the most common, caused by a blood clot that travels to the brain and blocks an artery. Getting treatment within three hours of the onset of symptoms with tissue plasminogen activator (tPA) medication can dissolve clots and can often lessen disability. Hemorrhagic strokes (not shown), caused when a blood vessel breaks and bleeds into the brain, account for 7 to 10 percent of strokes. More than half are fatal.

While strokes can and do occur at any age, nearly three-quarters of all strokes occur in people over the age of 65, and the risk of having a stroke more than doubles each decade between ages 55 and 85.

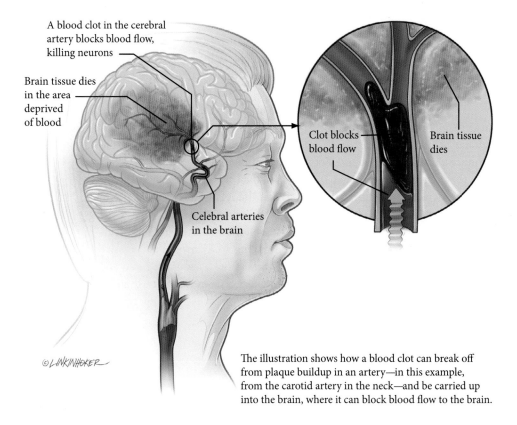

A blood clot in the cerebral artery blocks blood flow, killing neurons

Brain tissue dies in the area deprived of blood

Celebral arteries in the brain

Clot blocks blood flow

Brain tissue dies

©LINKINHOKER

The illustration shows how a blood clot can break off from plaque buildup in an artery—in this example, from the carotid artery in the neck—and be carried up into the brain, where it can block blood flow to the brain.

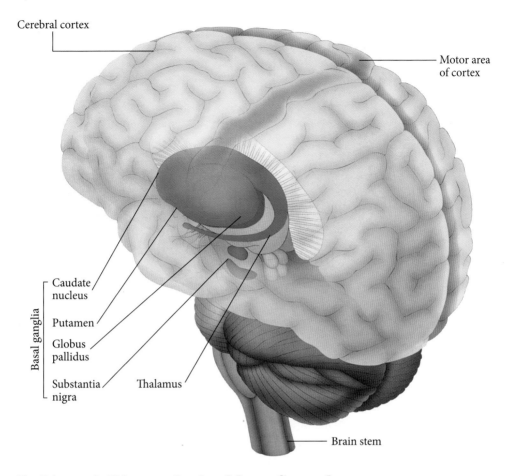

Cerebral cortex

Motor area of cortex

Basal ganglia

Caudate nucleus

Putamen

Globus pallidus

Substantia nigra

Thalamus

Brain stem

Parkinson's Disease: Losing Motor Control

Most cell death underlying Parkinson's disease occurs in a part of the brain called the substantia nigra, which controls voluntary movement and helps to regulate mood. Although the rest of the brain can compensate for this loss at first, when 50 to 80 percent of the cells in the substantia nigra have been lost, it can no longer carry on. At that point, other parts of the brain engaged in motor control, including the rest of the basal ganglia, the thalamus, and the cerebral cortex, can no longer work together, and movement becomes disjointed and uncontrollable

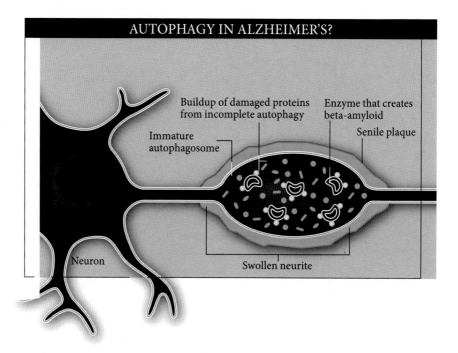

AUTOPHAGY IN ALZHEIMER'S?

Buildup of damaged proteins from incomplete autophagy

Enzyme that creates beta-amyloid

Senile plaque

Immature autophagosome

Neuron

Swollen neurite

When the Cleaning Stops

Your brain is constantly cleaning house to remove damaged proteins and other worn-out bits that clog up your neurons and contribute to swelling in the neurites that project from brain cells. But in an aging brain, the autophagosomes that gobble up neural garbage may not completely develop and instead become part of the trash. Enzymes (yellow) that create protein fragments called beta-amyloid seem to concentrate on these immature autophagosomes. These fragments collect on the outside of neurons (orange) and form the so-called senile plaques characteristic of brains with Alzheimer's disease, suggesting that poor neural housekeeping may contribute to dementia.

Brain Shrinkage in Alzheimer's Disease

As Alzheimer's disease progresses, brain cells die, and patients and family begin to notice memory and other cognitive lapses. It becomes possible to see signs of disease with brain imaging: Cell death shrinks the brain in areas that involve memory (the hippocampus) and higher-level brain functions (the cortex) and can be tracked with a form of magnetic resonance imaging (MRI) that measures brain volume. As the shrinkage accelerates, it ultimately involves many areas of the brain. Positron emission tomography (PET) scans can show increasing accumulations of beta-amyloid, marked by a tracer called PIBIB in the brain's frontal lobes. It increases over the course of two years even while the person remained cognitively normal.

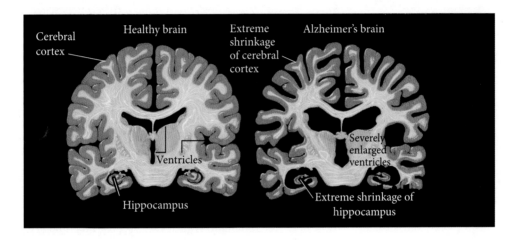

New Tools Detect Silent Early Signs of Dementia

The damaging processes underlying Alzheimer's disease start years before symptoms show up that would lead to a diagnosis. Researchers can now track it in living patients with tools—including brain imaging and spinal fluid tests that monitor Alzheimer's-related biomarkers—that detect signs of biological changes (such as mounting levels of toxic proteins) that routinely occur in the course of the disease. Researchers hope that one day biomarker testing will identify incipient disease in people and that treatment in this early stage will delay or prevent dementia.

Amyloid Accretion: Five to twenty years before diagnosis of Alzheimer's dementia

Early on, a protein fragment called beta-amyloid clumps up in the brain centers that form new memories. The amyloid buildup, a biomarker detected by the presence of plaques, damages synapses, the interface between neurons (detail). Amyloid blocks chemical signals from neurotransmitters from reaching receptors on receiving neurons. This buildup can be seen in various types of neuroimaging, including positron-emission tomography (PET), that detect a radioactive compound, Pittsburgh imaging compound-B (PIB), which is able to bind specifically to amyloid. A spinal tap can also gauge the amyloid biomarker.

Tau Buildup: One to five years before diagnosis

Before symptoms would substantiate an Alzheimer's diagnosis, a protein called tau inside neurons begins misbehaving. Normally tau helps to maintain the structure of tiny tubes (microtubules) critical to the proper functioning of neurons. But now phosphate groups begin to accumulate on tau proteins (detail), which detach from the microtubules. The tubules go on to disintegrate, and tau then aggregates, forming tangles that interfere with cellular functions. A sample of spinal fluid can detect this process.

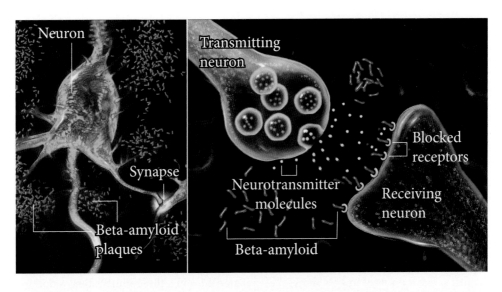

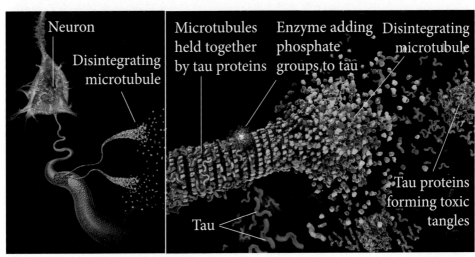

How Exercise Helps Your Brain Health: Walking May Slow Progression of Dementia

Researchers know that the volume of both the hippocampus and the medial temporal lobe shrink with age, beginning in late adulthood, and that this shrinkage is associated with impaired memory and increased risk for dementia. They also know that these areas are larger in more highly fit adults and that exercise benefits body and brain.

Now studies show that just plain walking can make your brain not only better but also bigger, especially in the areas important for memory, learning, and attention—and this is true for both those with normal aging brains and those with cognitive impairment. A study compared the effects of walking to a stretching routine. At the end of a year, MRIs showed the walking group slightly increased the volume of the hippocampus, while those who did a stretching routine showed no such growth. In fact, they lost volume in their hippocampus.

These figures show, in red and yellow, the beneficial effects of physical activity on the brains of healthy aging individuals and those with either mild cognitive impairment or Alzheimer's. The top row of images shows these relationships in a three-dimensional rendering of the brain, while the bottom row shows the prefrontal cortex findings in side-view cutaway images. The impaired brain shows more colored areas because these brains had more benefit from walking than healthy brains.

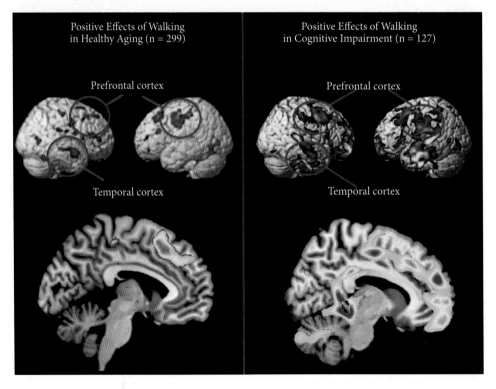

exercising your body. Several studies have already shown that exercise and socialization in later life have positive effects on the brain, and both of these are as easy as taking a walk and calling a friend. Even the simple act of practicing juggling for a week increases gray matter in brain areas involved in visual and motor activity (even if you never become very good at juggling).

What, then, is the rationale for using expensive brain games, which are essentially solitary activities that require you to shell out the bucks, sit on your gluteus maximus, stare at a screen, and exercise little more than your index finger as it pushes the button on the mouse? The immediate answer is that we don't know, because no one has done those sorts of scientific comparisons. So far, the exact type of most effective brain exercise remains undetermined. But perhaps both the hype and the promise, combined with a little personal financial investment, is just what you need to find the right motivation to train your brain in a systematic manner.

One thing remains clear: there's no serious harm to brain training other than the effect on your wallet (and the risk of some egg on your face if your 7-year-old granddaughter can play them better than you can).

Evidence is accumulating that some of them do not only improve the skills they are designed to help but likely generalize to other cognitive abilities and have some long-lasting benefits. And they are convenient packages that integrate training from many areas. If you're working at them now, keep it up. If you want to try one, start by taking advantage of the many free trial offers online to see what works best for you. What matters most is whether it challenges you at the right level and whether you enjoy using one enough to actually do it. But while you're at it, don't substitute computer games for physical exercise: that's an area where the scientific evidence for brain benefit is very strong.

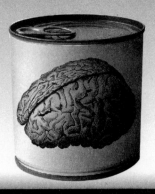

CHAPTER NINE

Nutrition
Fuel for Thought

Yes, there really is such a thing as brain food, and it isn't just fish (as your mom may have told you, although wild salmon heads the list).

What we eat, when, and how much affects not only our overall health and well-being but also our ability to think and our emotional stability, studies show. Mental slip-ups and slowdowns are a part of aging, but we may be able to prevent, ease, or delay some of them by paying attention to diet. Nutrients in foods—or a lack of them—can influence memory, learning, concentration, and decision making and even our risks of Alzheimer's and Parkinson's diseases.

Most of us know the basics about healthful eating: avoid saturated fats and transfats, processed meats, and simple carbohydrates; limit red meat; pile on the fruits, veggies, complex carbohydrates, grains, and nuts. Now ongoing research is showing us more specifics about brain-friendly foods.

Some basic facts: your brain needs fuel, and it needs it on a regular basis. Although it makes up a mere 2 percent of our body weight, it uses 20 percent of the body's metabolic fuel at rest.

Glucose is a major source of energy for most cells, including those in your brain. The brain operates best when blood glucose levels

---

PROVISIONS FOR BRAIN POWER

A well-balanced diet benefits the brain just as it does the body. This table highlights examples of the best brain foods (in **bold** type) and describes the functions of other nutrients found in foods that can influence concentration, memory, learning, and the overall health of the brain.

Nutrient	Function	Presence in Foods
Carbohydrates	Supply glucose for energy	Whole grains, fruits (especially **apples**), vegetables
Liquids	Stabilize circulation and nutrient transport, among other functions	Water, mineral water, unsweetened herbal and fruit teas
Caffeine, in small amounts	Dilates the blood vessels in the brain; increases concentration and memory	Coffee, black tea, **green tea**
Iron	Transports oxygen	Red meats, pumpkin seeds, sesame, soy flour, millet, poppy seeds, pine nuts, wheat germ, **oats**, dill, parsley, yeast, spinach, watercress, lentils, soybeans, white beans

Nutrient	Function	Presence in Foods
Calcium	Conducts neural signals	Milk and milk products, poppy seeds, figs, sesame, soybeans, legumes, **nuts**, whole grains, wheat germ, oatmeal, broccoli, watercress, green vegetables, parsley
Zinc	Aids many chemical reactions in the brain; important for concentration and memory	Wheat germ, poppy seeds, figs, sesame seeds, pumpkin seeds, meat, eggs, milk, cheese, fish, carrots, whole grain bread, potatoes
Phenylalanine, tyrosine	Act as precursors of epinephrine, norepinephrine, and dopamine; important for concentration and memory	**Fish** (tuna, trout), meat, milk products, **soybeans**, cheese (cottage cheese), peanuts, wheat germ, almonds
Serine, methionine	Act as precursors of acetylcholine; essential for learning and memory formation	**Fish**, turkey, chicken, soybeans, beef, cashews, wheat germ, broccoli, peas, spinach, whole grain bread, rice
Vitamin B$_1$ (thiamine)	Enables glucose metabolism; aids nerve cell function	Whole grains (wheat, spelt), oatmeal, wheat germ, sunflower seeds, legumes, nuts, pork
Unsaturated fatty acids, including omega-3 fatty acids	Build cell membranes	**Fish**, walnuts, spinach, corn oil, peanut oil, soybean oil, grape seed oil, flax seed

SOURCE: "Brain Food," *Scientific American Mind*, Oct.–Nov. 2007.

are stable. Very high levels (hyperglycemia, such as with diabetes) interfere with mental function, and so do very low levels (hypoglycemia, when blood sugar drops). In a 2005 study, psychologist Daniel J. Cox and his colleagues at the University of Virginia Health System found that about half of the 230 people with diabetes they were monitoring were slower and less accurate at basic verbal and math tasks when their glucose levels rose above a certain threshold. The scientists speculate this happens because it alters the structure of blood vessels at the blood-brain barrier or by triggering changes in the production of neurotransmitters, the chemical messengers in the brain.

Eating complex carbohydrates rather than simple sugars can help stabilize glucose concentrations and guard against mental lapses. Studies also indicate that protein-packed fare seems to boost attention. Your brain is dependent on amino acids, the building blocks of proteins, for producing essential neurochemicals: the amino acid tyrosine, for example, is needed to make epinephrine and dopamine, both of which contribute to alertness.

A boost in these amino acids could partly explain why small high-protein meals featuring low-fat dairy products, fish, lean meats, and legumes may make people more alert and attentive, as some studies have shown. Protein may also boost attention by stabilizing blood glucose levels. In a 2002 study of fifteen healthy male students who ate meals with differing ratios of carbohydrate to protein, nutrition scientist Karina Fischer of the Swiss Federal Institute of Technology in Zurich and her colleagues found that relative to a carbohydrate-rich meal, balanced and protein-rich meals led to more accurate short-term memory and improved attention beginning one hour after eating.

Minerals and vitamins are vital. Iron, for example, is important for staying mentally sharp: it chaperones vital oxygen to the brain, and deficiencies cause anemia, which has been connected with cognitive decline and Alzheimer's. The right kinds of fats—omega-3 fatty acids found in fish and some nut and plant oils—oil our mental gears and protect our heart health.

When we eat is also important for brain function. Since your brain can't store carbohydrates, it requires a constant supply of glucose. When blood glucose drops, our faculties fade and we lose the ability to concentrate. To stay mentally sharp, it's best to eat breakfast and then small meals or snacks throughout the day.

How much we eat, researchers have found, affects brain health, giving overweight people in their 40s yet another reason to shed pounds before their elder years: obesity in midlife elevates the risk of developing Alzheimer's disease. Researchers at the Kaiser Permanente Foundation Research Institute in Oakland, California, charted more than ten thousand people for up to thirty years beyond their 40s. The heavier people were, the more likely they were to develop dementia. In fact, people who were obese in midlife were 74 percent more likely to have dementia, and overweight people were 35 percent more likely.

Finally, it could be how you eat as well. At least one interesting study shows that the mere act of chewing can improve memory. Cognitive neuroscientist Lucy Wilkinson and her coworkers at the University of Northumbria reported in 2002 that subjects who chewed sugar-free gum were better able to remember words than subjects who did not chew anything, perhaps because chewing improves blood flow to brain areas that are important for memory. Who knew?

Glucose Is Not So Sweet to the Brain

Your glucose balance is tricky, and as we grow older, it becomes more so since our bodies become less adept at metabolizing glucose in the bloodstream. A study has linked these rising levels with momentary forgetfulness, pinpointing exactly where in the brain the aging process acts—a finding that could help ward off memory lapses.

High blood levels of glucose could contribute to senior moments, those pesky instances of not-so-total recall—forgetting where we left our reading glasses, or what we did last weekend, or, of course and seemingly always, where those darned keys are.

The nature of senior moments has led scientists to believe they stem from disruptions in the hippocampus—an area that, among other roles, acts as the brain's "save" button, allowing us to retain new information. Using functional magnetic resonance imaging, Scott Small, a neurologist at Columbia University, and colleagues looked at the effects of increased blood glucose in the hippocampus of 181 people aged 65 or older with no history of dementia. They found that elevated levels impaired the function of a section of the hippocampus called the dentate gyrus, a hot spot of age-related impairment.

But here's the good news: blood glucose is not alone in selectively affecting dentate gyrus performance. Small shows that exercise improves its function in both mice and humans. The newer research, he points out, suggests that these positive effects may actually result from the influence of regular exercise on the body's ability to break down and use glucose.

Psychiatrist Mony de Leon of New York University explains that the new study "may be showing a very fundamental aging process that might have some reversibility built into it." If you correct glucose imbalances, he says, you may be able to forget about forgetfulness.

And also remember that we need glucose—in small amounts, from complex carbohydrates—to keep alert. It's the quantity we need to worry about. And if you've already forgotten about the many good effects of exercise, turn back to Chapter Eight.

Forget the Fructose

Fructose, another sugar, is believed to be worse for the body and brain than glucose.

Also called fruit sugar, it comes from many vegetables and fruits, including sugarcane, sugar beets, and corn. The problem appears to come from the levels of high-fructose corn syrups used in many commercially produced foods, from breakfast cereals to beverages: it's been blamed for part of the obesity epidemic. Research with overweight people and sweetened beverages has shown more insulin resistance and other risk factors for heart disease and diabetes when fructose made up 25 percent of calories compared to glucose-sweetened beverages.

In animals, fructose-rich diets increase the production of fat and promote resistance to the energy-regulating hormone insulin. New research suggests that memory suffers as well, at least in rats.

Neuroscientist Marise B. Parent of Georgia State University and her colleagues fed eleven adolescent rats a diet in which fructose supplied 60 percent of the calories. For ten other rats, cornstarch took the place of the sweetener. The scientists trained the rats to find a submerged platform in a pool. Two days after the training ended, Parent's group removed the pool's platform and recorded where the rats, now adults, swam. The cornstarch group spent most of its time around the platform's old location, but the fructose-fed rats visited this area significantly less often. They can learn the platform's location, Parent notes, but they can't remember it for long periods. Another research group has shown in hamsters that insulin resistance can affect the hippocampus.

We can often get a sugar double whammy in the typical human diet: fructose and glucose are often used together, and the body metabolizes each sugar differently. People tend to consume both sweeteners at the same time, as high-fructose corn syrup (which is most commonly 55 percent fructose and 45 percent glucose) in many foods and table sugar (half fructose and half glucose), and glucose aids the body's absorption of fructose. Glucose and fructose occur naturally together in fruit, for example. All foods have some glucose, which is good. Those with the highest amounts that could boost your blood level to a unhealthy level include all sugars (and, yes, honey counts) and foods with sugars. These are too numerous to list but include condiments, alcohol, most soft drinks, simple carbohydrates like pasta and white bread, fruit juices, and many fruits.

Omega-3, the Essential Oil

Your brain needs oils and fats to function, but they need to be the right kind. There's been a plethora of good news about omega-3 oils, found in cold-water fish and flax seed and added to many foods such as the eggs of some specially fed chickens. The omega-3 fatty acids are made up of three kinds of oils. Fish oil contains both docosahexaenoic acid (DHA) and eicosapentaenoic acid (EPA), while some nut (English walnuts) and vegetable oils (canola, soybean, flaxseed/linseed, olive) contain alpha-linolenic acid (ALA).

Rightly famous for aiding heart health (statistics show that eating as few as one to three portions of coldwater fish per month significantly decreases the risk of stroke), the polyunsaturated omega-3 fatty acids can oil your mental gears as well.

Omega-3 also could relieve anxiety and inflammation, both conditions bad for the brain. A recent study with fish oil supplements showed a marked reduction in both inflammation and anxiety among a cohort of healthy young people, so elderly brains might benefit even more because both anxiety and inflammation increase risks for Alzheimer's and other dementias. The dose used was about 2.5 grams of omega-3 per day, in this formula: 2,085 milligrams of eicosapentaenoic acid (EPA) plus 348 mg of docosahexaenoic acid (DHA).

Some studies comparing the occurrence of Alzheimer's disease between elderly persons with different levels of dietary omega-3 suggest that risk of Alzheimer's is significantly lower among those with higher levels of fish and omega-3 consumption. However, since these were not randomized controlled trials, they don't definitively prove omega-3 reduces Alzheimer's risk.

Found in coldwater fish such as mackerel, tuna, herring, and salmon, the fish-derived oils are components of nerve cell membranes and myelin, and they help to keep blood vessels in the brain healthy at any age, from fetal on to the end. Other good oils are flax (the best plant-based source of omega-3), linseed, canola, soy, and walnut oils, which contain significant quantities of alpha-linolenic acid, a shorter-chain fat that the body converts into long-chain omega-3 fatty acids. Olive oil rates right up there as well. A recent French study of the medical records of 7,625 healthy people ages 65 and older from three cities in France (Bordeaux, Dijon, and Montpellier) found that those who regularly used olive oil for cooking and as salad dressing had a 41 percent lower risk of stroke compared to those who never used olive oil in their diet.

Three cautions: Avoid using these plant oils for frying or sautéing on high heat because high heat turns them into transfatty acids, which may have detrimental effects on learning and overall health. If you want to take an omega-3 supplement, read the labels carefully: it should contain EPA and DHA. Finally, talk to your doctor before taking these (or any other supplement) because omega-3 supplements are blood thinners and can cause excess bleeding, particularly in people taking anticoagulant drugs.

Your Brain on Berries, Chocolate, and Wine: The Flavonoid Connection

Chemical compounds common in most of the foods your mom urged you to eat (and some you may consider indulgences) can shore up memory, boost brain power, and perhaps protect against Alzheimer's and Parkinson's diseases.

Flavonoids, chemicals naturally found in foods as diverse as berries, tofu, tea, dark chocolate, and red wine, act as antioxidants and can improve memory, learning, and general cognitive function, including reasoning skills, decision making, verbal comprehension, and numerical ability. They may, some studies suggest, help slow the decline in mental facility often seen with aging. In some studies, they even appeared to reverse memory loss.

Flavonoids protect cells from damage caused by the ubiquitous unstable molecules known as free radicals, the rogue chemicals formed by our own bodies during metabolism and also spawned by pollution, cigarette smoke, and radiation. As a result, researchers have for decades investigated the potential of these compounds for boosting immunity, staving off cancer, and reducing excess inflammation; flavonoids also appear to help regulate blood flow and blood pressure. Now we find that a brain boost may come from interactions between flavonoids and proteins vital to brain cell structure and function, changing the chemistry of neurons for the better. They may also boost and regulate levels of enzymes called kinases, which are essential to learning and memory.

It's easy to add them to your diet—perhaps a wee bit too easy if you tend to overindulge in wine and chocolate. To date, scientists have identified more than six thousand different flavonoids that come in a variety of types in foods, including berries, fruits, vegetables, and cereal grains.

Animal studies showed that middle-aged rodents that ate foods rich in flavonoids performed better than their peers fed the usual diet,

FLAVORS OF FLAVONOIDS

Scientists have discovered thousands of different flavonoids. Flavonoids come in several subgroups, shown with their most common food sources here:

Flavonoid Group	Example Compounds	Food Sources
Flavonols	Quercetin, kaempferol	Spinach, peppers, onions
Flavones	Luteolin, apigenin	Parsley, celery
Flavanones	Eriodictyol, epicatechin	Tea, cocoa, wine
Anthocyandins	Cyanidin, peonidin	Berries, grapes, wine
Isoflavones	Genistein, daidzein	Soy foods such as tofu

and they performed better at the end of the study than at the beginning. Meanwhile, studies of humans were showing that eating meals full of flavonoids might have brain benefits. In a study published in 2007 epidemiologist Luc Letenneur and his colleagues at the Institut National de la Santé et de la Recherche Médicale in France asked 1,640 cognitively healthy older adults to fill out a questionnaire about their dietary habits and take a test of their cognitive function over a period of ten years. They repeated the questionnaire and test four times during that decade, correlating diet information with their cognitive test scores.

The researchers found that those with the highest levels of flavonoid intake at the start of the study also performed best on thinking skills such as the ability to do simple arithmetic, recall items in different categories, repeat words and phrases, and identify time and place. And their performance tended to be more stable over time than that of those with very low levels of flavonoids in their diet, whose thinking skills tended to decline over time. Those with the best scores were eating between 18 and 37 milligrams of flavonoids a day, which translates to (as one example) about fifteen blueberries, a quarter of a cup of orange juice, and half a cup of tofu.

Moreover, specific compounds have shown specific positive results—and that includes tea (black and green and even decaffeinated), wine, and dark chocolate. A 2009 research team, led by nutritionist Eha Nurk at the University of Oslo in Norway, asked two thousand adults in their early 70s to fill out food-frequency questionnaires and then tested them on measures of mental agility. Those who reported regular consumption of wine, tea, and chocolate, which are especially rich in flavonoids, performed significantly better than those who consumed these items only rarely.

Dark chocolate's heart-healthy ability may be part of the reason: a recent study shows that cocoa, the main ingredient in chocolate, appears to reduce the risk of heart disease by boosting levels of high-density lipoprotein (HDL), or "good" cholesterol, and decreasing levels of low-density lipoprotein (LDL), or "bad" cholesterol. It also makes some of us feel better. Chocolate contains theobromine, a substance that has an effect similar to but milder than caffeine, and phenylethylamine, a mild mood elevator. It's said that Jeanne Calment, the world's longest-lived person to date, ate two pounds of chocolate per week.

A TIPPLE A DAY IS GOOD FOR YOUR BRAIN

Heavy drinking is bad for just about every part of you, but numerous studies have shown a daily drink seems to prop up memory and cognitive function.

A recent analysis of 143 studies from the Loyola University Chicago Stritch School of Medicine adds even more weight to the value of moderate social drinking, especially wine. Researchers reviewed studies dating to 1977 that included more than 365,000 participants in nineteen countries. In fourteen of the countries, including the United States, they found that moderate drinkers—one drink per day for women, two for men—were 23 percent less likely to develop cognitive impairment or Alzheimer's disease and other forms of dementia than those who didn't drink alcohol at all. They also found no difference between men and women as to the effects of alcohol, and the protective effect held up after adjusting for age, education, and smoking.

Another study, this one from Wake Forest University Baptist Medical Center, compared teetotalers with light, moderate, and heavy drinkers over a six-year period. It found that moderate drinkers (eight to fourteen drinks per week) who started the study with no cognitive problems were 37 percent less likely to develop Alzheimer's disease compared to abstainers. However, those who had some mild cognitive loss or who were heavy drinkers, or both, had a faster decline.

Researchers don't know why moderate alcohol drinking helps the brain. It's known to benefit the heart, raise HDLs, and improve blood flow to the brain. The study's coauthors, Edward J. Neafsey and Michael A. Collins, speculated that small amounts of alcohol stress brain cells and toughen them up so that they better cope with other dementia-related stressors.

The elders who did not consume any wine, tea, or chocolate scored worst of all—an effect, by the way, found in several studies. Individuals who reported drinking wine regularly (but in moderation) had about a 45 percent lower risk of poor cognitive performance, defined as a score in the lowest tenth percentile on the test. The benefit for tea or chocolate was a 10 to 20 percent diminished risk. Those who regularly consumed all three items decreased their chances of a poor score by 70 percent.

Another study found that blueberries boosted brain power in rodents as well as a small group of humans aged 75 or older who had mild memory loss, but it took a lot of those little berries. After consuming two cups of wild blueberry juice (the equivalent of five cups of blueberries a day) for twelve weeks, they performed 30 percent better on memory recall tests than a control group. In addition to flavonoids, blueberries also have healthy polyphenolics, another class of antioxidant, found in many natural foods such as grapes, acai, and strawberries.

Soy isoflavones may improve memory by acting like weak estrogens, binding to and stimulating estrogen receptors on neurons. Exciting these receptors is known to trigger changes in both neuronal shape and chemistry in the hippocampus, whose function most likely diminishes with age. These changes may facilitate communication between neurons and thereby improve memory.

Researchers in recent years have tested the effects of adding flavonoids to people's diets, the human equivalent of the work with rats. Although it's hard to control people's base diets—humans aren't confined to one dining spot, all eating the same chow—adding flavonoids to your diet might preserve or improve memory, thought processing, and the whole cognitive shebang.

In 2009 nutrition researcher Anna Macready and her colleagues at the University of Reading in England reviewed fifteen small dietary intervention trials in which researchers tested this thesis by asking people to add flavonoid-containing foods to their meals. The findings

ANTIOXIDANTS MIGHT SLOW HEARING LOSS

It's the subject of many jokes—and woes—about aging: the loss of our formerly acute hearing. Forty percent of Americans older than age 65 suffer from hearing loss, and by 2030 some 65 million Americans will be hard of hearing.

Joint work by researchers at the Universities of Wisconsin, Florida, Washington, and Tokyo has now uncovered the mechanism behind some age-related hearing loss, and with the help of simple chemicals, they have managed to keep old mice hearing as well as young pups.

The team investigated free radicals, which harm cells in a process called oxidation. They've been implicated in many age-related maladies, from wrinkles to memory loss, but had not yet been tied to hearing loss. They found that cells stressed by oxidative damage release a protein called Bak, which triggers a cascade of events culminating in cell suicide. And unlike most other cells in the body, which are replaced with new cells as they die, the inner ear's sensory nerve cells and ganglion neurons do not regenerate, so hearing loss is permanent.

Researchers compared normal mice with genetically engineered mice that do not have the gene necessary to make Bak. The Bak-deficient mice didn't develop hearing problems as they aged, but the ordinary mice, subjected to the same oxidative stress, became hard of hearing. Searching for an intervention to stave off free radical damage, scientist found two antioxidants: alpha lipoic acid (found in organ meats and spinach, broccoli, and brewer's yeast) and coenzyme Q10 (present in many foods and abundant in meat, fish, and poultry). When fed these antioxidants, normal mice were protected from free radical damage in the cochlea. However, it's not known if this would help other kinds of hearing loss.

were complicated by inconsistencies in the types of cognitive testing, but the authors concluded that flavonoid consumption from any of the sources examined improved aspects of cognition such as verbal comprehension, simple reasoning and decision making, object recall, and recognition of numerical patterns. Flavonoids also seemed to hone fine motor skills such as finger tapping.

There's more. Some flavonoids may even spur the growth of new nerve cells in the hippocampus and defend neurons from damage and death, and so combat Alzheimer's and Parkinson's diseases. Animal and cell culture data suggest that flavonoids may offset the effects of glutamate—a neurotransmitter that at high concentrations damages neurons—by preventing these toxins from binding to receptors on neurons. Flavonoids also may oppose the action of some enzymes called secretases that are involved in beta-amyloid production (both positively and negatively) and that might be elevated in some neurodegenerative disorders.

Scientists don't yet know which flavonoid-containing foods have the greatest potential for bettering the brain, but eating flavonoid-rich foods is probably better than taking supplements. Processing may destroy or reduce the actual flavonoid content of supplements, and intact fruits and vegetables (rather than juice or supplements) are likely to contain the amounts and combinations of these compounds that are most beneficial to the brain.

You don't have to create an unusual daily diet. Following the current U.S. Department of Agriculture (USDA) dietary guidelines, which call for eating two cups of fruit and two and a half cups of vegetables every day, will ensure that you get a generous variety of these brain-boosting compounds.

And let's not forget water, the nectar of life: so simple, so available, so inexpensive and easy to ingest—and yet dehydration is an issue among the aging brains. Indeed, dehydration mimics dementia in the elderly. Nutrients can reach the brain in adequate amounts only if the body gets enough fluid. Studies have shown that even slight dehydration slows the rate at which nutrients can enter the brain, producing short-term memory deficits and reasoning difficulties, among other cognitive woes.

Caffeine: A Perk for Your Brain

The world's most consumed drug, coffee, has been praised and damned. The latest finding is that it can be good or bad for your brain, depending on how big a "dose" you're taking.

In small quantities, caffeinated beverages such as tea and coffee can improve short-term concentration and facilitate learning and memory. Some studies suggest that moderate amounts might even help protect against Alzheimer's and Parkinson's diseases (and tea also contains flavonoids). Caffeine perks up the brain, and because it removes chemical inhibitors from the brain's activity-regulating system (the reticular-activating system), it can put the brain into overdrive.

The effect of coffee takes hold within about twenty minutes and lasts for two to three hours. Tea has a weaker but longer-lasting impact because it contains less caffeine than coffee and its caffeine is released more slowly. But drink too much caffeine (four cups of coffee or more in a day), and your ability to concentrate will likely decline, studies suggest. After seven cups, you also might start hallucinating or suffer the physiological effects of stress, which provokes the release of cortisol and is not good for your brain (see "Maybe It's Not Alzheimer's Disease" in Chapter Four). It can also contribute to panic and anxiety attacks. And massive amounts, say, the equivalent of one hundred cups or several grams of caffeine taken in pills over a short period of time, could kill you.

The July 2009 *Journal of Alzheimer's Disease* reviewed two studies with mice bred to develop Alzheimer's disease that showed that caffeine significantly decreased levels of proteins connected with Alzheimer's.

There is some controversy about whether coffee is truly addictive, since it doesn't affect the dopamine pathways strongly, but don't stop cold turkey: you may bring on a headache.

Is There a Pill for That? Supplements and Vitamins

We're always looking for a magic potion or pill, which accounts for the enormous amount spent on substances such as herbs and other such supplements. But other than the vitamins suggested by your doctor, most supplements and herbs are unproven and probably a waste of money. More than one skeptical doctor has called supplement use "making expensive urine."

And rightly so. Extracts of ginkgo, for example, were widely touted for years as a memory aid. This may be the world's oldest tree, but, alas, results of a six-year study of old adults aged 72 to 96 found that taking 120 milligrams twice daily didn't result in any less cognitive loss. Others, such as St. John's wort, touted for depression and anxiety, has been found in numerous studies to have little good effect—and it can interfere with many prescription drugs.

Nevertheless, some supplements can help brain health. Researchers are finding, for example, that curcumin (turmeric), a spice used in curries, has been shown in test tubes to reduce beta-amyloid. A study showed that Chinese people who ate it in curry had improved cognitive scores, and Alzheimer's disease rates are the among lowest in the world in Asia, where turmeric is used in many foods eaten daily.

Vitamins, minerals, and trace elements are important for brain function, so a daily multivitamin is a good idea as we age. Even slight vitamin and mineral deficits—which may result, for example, from a diet of fast food—can lead to fatigue, forgetfulness, and concentration problems.

Iron is vital for brain function: researchers found that sixteen weeks of iron supplementation closed the intellectual gap for anemic women, improving their cognitive performance between five- and sevenfold. Vitamin C can aid iron absorption, so vegetarians can improve their iron intake by eating such foods (see the table earlier in this chapter for a list of them) in conjunction with iron-containing plant foods. Potassium, sodium, and calcium are used for nerve cell signaling and metabolic reactions in the brain. Vitamin B_1, in particular, enables glucose metabolism.

B vitamin deficiencies are notorious for mimicking dementia. Now researchers are finding that large doses of B-complex vitamins could reduce the rate of brain shrinkage by half in elderly people with memory problems and slow the progression of dementia. A two-year clinical trial in Oxford, England, involving 271 men over the age of 70 with mild cognitive impairment, has shown that B vitamins, including daily doses of 20 milligrams of B_6, .5 milligrams of B_{12}, and .8 milligrams of folic acid, slowed the progress. Magnetic resonance imaging scans taken before and after the study showed differences in brain shrinkage.

Gustavo C. Román, medical director of the Alzheimer and Dementia Center at the Methodist Neurological Institute in Houston, said that patients who already exhibit signs of dementia and test positive for high levels of homocysteine are more likely to respond well to large doses of B vitamins: he may prescribe weekly injections of B_{12} for four weeks and then high oral doses of folic acid, B_6, and B_{12}. Homocysteine is an amino acid in the blood, and high blood levels are linked to an increased risk of developing Alzheimer's disease.

Your brain might also need more vitamin D, a common deficiency in older people. Vitamin D is well known for promoting bone health, but scientists have found that this fat-soluble nutrient is vital for brain health as well—and, ironically, the push to prevent skin cancer may have unwittingly contributed to impaired brain function.

D, the "sunshine vitamin," is synthesized in our skin when it is exposed to direct sunlight, but sunblock impedes this process. And since many older folks avoid the sun or participate less in outdoor activities, D deficiencies are more likely with aging and could hasten cognitive problems.

Two European studies looked at vitamin D and cognitive function. The first, led by neuroscientist David Llewellyn of the University of Cambridge, assessed vitamin D levels in more than seventeen hundred men and women from England, aged 65 or older. Subjects were divided into four groups based on vitamin D blood levels, from severely low to optimum. The scientists found that the lower the subjects' vitamin D levels, the more negative their performance was on a battery of mental tests—and those in the lowest group were more than twice as likely to be cognitively impaired.

A second study, led by scientists at the University of Manchester in England, looked at vitamin D levels and cognitive performance in more than thirty-one hundred men aged 40 to 79 in eight countries across Europe and found that people with lower vitamin D levels had slower information processing speed, especially men older than 60 years.

So how much is enough vitamin D? Forget those USDA recommendations of 400 IU (international units) daily. Experts say we need 1,000 to 2,000 IU daily—about the amount your body will synthesize from fifteen to thirty minutes of sun exposure two to three times a week. You may need more if you are deficient, so ask your doctor about a test for D levels.

But do remember: anything strong enough to help you can also hurt you, especially when taken in large doses and in combination with other supplements and medicines. A common problem is excessive bleeding from ingesting several drugs and supplements that have anticoagulant or blood-thinning effects. So be sure to consult your doctor before taking any supplements, and check that your medical records include a notation on everything you are putting into your body and brain.

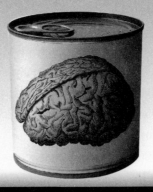

CHAPTER TEN

The Social Treatment

Sometimes it seems that everything the doctor orders for good health can be painful, unpleasant, or just plain boring.

But there's one prescription that is downright enjoyable for most of us and might just help preserve your brain: socializing. Having and using a social network, primarily the face-to-face kind, has been found to extend life and the quality of life and is associated with reduced risks of dementia and other ailments.

In fact, research has found that the good effects of companionship, romantic and otherwise, are so profound that an active social life may be the next prescription from your doctor. In the not-too-distant future, he or she may tell you, "Find two more friends, and call me in the morning."

More than one hundred years of research shows that having a healthy social life is vital to staying mentally and physically healthy. Overall, social support increases survival by some 50 percent, and having real-life and complex social networks increased survival rates by 91 percent, concluded the authors behind a new meta-analysis covering more than 300,000 participants across all ages.

"I don't think a lot of people recognize that our relationships can have a physical impact as well as emotional," says Julianne Holt-Lunstad, an associate psychology professor at Brigham Young University and coauthor of the study.

Social support has been linked to lower blood pressure, and a diverse collection of contacts is associated with better immune system functioning. The list continues to grow, now encompassing other bodily processes such as wound healing and inflammation.

In fact, feeling lonely can trigger bodily changes known to be bad for your brain. The initial results of a University of California, Los Angeles, study found that people who scored in the top 15 percent of a psychiatric questionnaire for measuring loneliness showed increased gene activity linked to inflammation and reduced gene activity associated with antibody production and antiviral responses. Patterns of gene expression were specifically related to the brain's feelings of loneliness, not to other negative feelings such as depression.

In a study of 1,023 Taiwanese adults, researcher Steven Cole analyzed data from a range of lonely people and found that the stress hormone cortisol was not doing its job of suppressing the genes associated with inflammation. Inflammation is a known risk factor for dementia and a variety of serious illnesses that contribute to it, such as heart disease. Recent animal studies from Cole's group confirm the link: cortisol receptors stopped working in rhesus monkeys that were socially stressed.

And socializing protects your brain. Harvard School of Public Health researchers found evidence that elderly people in the United

States who have an active social life may have a slower rate of memory decline. Using the Health and Retirement Study report of 2008, they examined data from more than sixteen thousand older people over a six-year period, testing memory and recall. They found memory did decline somewhat overall, but it declined twice as fast among those who were the least integrated socially (and most among those with fewer than twelve years of education). A Kaiser Permanente study of 2,249 women 78 or older found the same positive connection between social networks and brain health.

More recently, a 2011 Rush University study of 1,138 older folks with a mean age of 80 found that those who were the most socially active had one-quarter the cognitive decline of the least social. They measured social activity through a questionnaire that asked about social interactions such as going to restaurants and sporting events, taking trips with friends, visiting relatives, doing volunteer work, attending religious services, and even participating in off-track betting. They measured cognitive function using a battery of memory and other tests.

None of the study participants had any signs of cognitive impairment at the start of the study, but over an average of five years, the gap widened between those with the highest levels of social activity and the least socially active. And this was true when checked for variables that might have accounted for cognitive decline, such as age, exercise, and health.

You've Got a Friend, We Hope

The benefit of friends, family, and even colleagues turns out to be just as good for long-term survival as giving up a fifteen-cigarette-a-day smoking habit, the Holt-Lunstad study found. And by the study's numbers, interpersonal social networks are more crucial to physical health than exercising or beating obesity.

Researchers have been surprised to learn that friendships increased life expectancy to a far greater extent than, say, frequent contact with children and other relatives. This benefit held even after these friends had moved away to another area and was independent of factors such as socioeconomic status, health, and way of life.

Loneliness and isolation are bad for our brains as well as our bodies. University of Chicago psychologist John Cacioppo, who has been studying social isolation as it affects the brain and our other biology, finds it disconcertingly associated with illness, mental and physical. He finds lonely people take more risks, are more impulsive, and eat more comfort (and unhealthy) food. Those who feel disconnected from others live with a low level threat feeling, among other ills. That stress contributes to higher blood pressure, and we know that what's bad for the heart is bad for the brain.

What exactly underlies this effect on longevity and brain health? Apparently, the scientists posit, it is not merely the mutual buoying of spirits that occurs among associates. What's more important is that the support given and received by friends is voluntary and pleasurable and not just the result of a sense of duty or convention. We may not be able to choose our families, as the saying goes, but we can choose our friends.

Having relationships with people to whom we are important has a positive effect on physical and mental health. It lowers stress and the tendency toward depression, along with tendencies to unhealthy habits such as smoking and drinking (depending on your friends' habits, of course). Long-time friends knew us then as well as now; newer friends offer fresh perspectives. In times of calamity in particular, our support networks can raise our mood and feelings of self-worth and offer helpful strategies for dealing with a personal challenge.

Taking a trip to visit long-time but distant friends, a leisurely lunch with old friends, or a night out with buddies who share your interests might be just what the doctor ordered. Sometimes we view these events as a distraction from other healthy habits, such as going to the gym or getting a good night's sleep, or decide it's just too darn much trouble. It also costs money (and a growing amount of discomfort and hassle) to travel. But maintaining old friendships is a good investment in your health.

Previous research has pointed to happiness as a key to longevity, but apparently our relationships don't even have to be good to boost our health. In most of the studies, social connections weren't classified in terms of their quality. Most likely negative associations were lumped in with positive ones. This means the benefit of positive social connections is likely to be even higher.

Talk to Teens, Live Longer

"Youth is a wonderful thing," George Bernard Shaw once said. "What a crime to waste it on children."

FIVE GREAT THINGS SOCIALIZING DOES FOR YOUR BRAIN

Friendship is a great investment for brain and body. It helps lift your spirits, and that includes relationships with your animal friends. Consider these benefits:

1. Lowers your blood pressure and inflammation, and thus heart disease and risk of stroke and other brain damage
2. Improves your immune system functioning, lowering risks from disease that could harm your brain
3. Helps you take better care of your health (for the ones you love, if not for yourself)
4. Lowers or delays your risk of memory loss or Alzheimer's disease by keeping your brain active
5. Relieves pain; just holding hands with someone you care about lowers pain perception

Indeed. But recent research suggests that youthful energy may not be "wasted" after all. Through social interactions, the young can pass some of their vigor on to the elderly, improving an older generation's cognitive abilities and vascular health and even increasing the life span.

Sharon Arkin, a psychiatrist at the University of Arizona, runs a clinical program in which Alzheimer's patients engage in exercise sessions with college students. She showed that her program stabilizes cognitive decline and improves patients' moods.

Researchers who have also documented these benefits in mammals such as rats, guinea pigs, and nonhuman primates haven't been sure why youth is a tonic. Biologist Chun-Fang Wu of the University of Iowa and then-graduate student Hongyu Ruan offer a genetic explanation. They found that the presence of youthful, active fruit flies doubled the life span of a group of flies with a mutation in Sod1, a gene that has been linked in humans to Alzheimer's disease and amyotrophic lateral sclerosis, a motor-neuron disorder also known as Lou Gehrig's disease.

Fruit flies are quite social, and social cues govern both their reproduction and aging process—and their genes are easier to manipulate than those of their mammalian counterparts. By altering SOD1, Wu created flies that died after only about two weeks, a quarter of their normal life span. When housed with younger flies, however, the SOD1 mutants lived for about thirty days and became more physically fit, according to heat stress tests and other measures.

Wu thinks it is possible the SOD1 gene could be playing a part in the human body as well. Besides the gene's association with ALS (and somewhat with Alzheimer's), Wu found that flies with the SOD1 mutation were more receptive to social cues than flies with other age-accelerating mutations.

While we're waiting for further studies to determine the therapeutic potential of intergenerational socialization, it won't hurt to spend more time with those teenage grandkids—maybe at the gym or in the park.

Finding and Making Friends in Later Life

Being socially involved improves cognition in general and seems to help thwart the arrival of dementia. Yet it's not as easy in later life to make friends as it was when we were younger and were connected through school, work, and children's activities. It takes some courage to get out there in an unfamiliar place, put forth a friendly smile, and possibly face rejection. But there are still plenty of ways to meet and get to know people. Psychologists, self-help writers, and successful socializers offer tips on where and how to friend (to use the verb form of today). Here's a summary of some practical advice:

1. *Show up, and pay attention.* Accept all invitations (within reason), even the one for your second cousin's grandson's graduation party. Attend art gallery openings, fundraising events, community celebrations—even if you have to go alone. Check out neighborhood yard sales (and the neighbors). You can't meet people if you don't get out. And the more you do it, the easier it gets to make friends.

2. *Join a group, take a class, volunteer.* Take a course, join a gym or tai chi course, sign up for a lecture series, find a walking group, or volunteer at the library, local animal shelter, museum, or other nonprofit. There are many social groups connected to church. If you haven't been a churchgoer, check out a nondenominational group such as the Unitarian Universalists. Soon you'll be seeing the same people week after week, and friendly encounters will follow.

3. *Befriend friends of friends.* Someone you like a lot probably has friends you'll also like. Invite them and a friend to join you for an event or for lunch or dinner and a movie or a play. Tell friends you are looking to expand your social circle.

4. *Use the Internet, but wisely.* If you haven't entered cyberspace, try it out. The Internet offers endless possibilities for connection with old friends and new. The number of those who have reconnected

after decades is legion, and friends halfway around the globe can be in instant communication. With a camera in your computer, you can even videophone others with Skype for free (at least for now), whether they are in Topeka or Timbuktu. But beware of disconnecting from the real world. It's easy for online and virtual relationships to take the place of real contact. If you are too hooked into cyberspace, turn off and tune in only now and then. Use your computer to find local activities, make plans, and stay in touch, but not as a substitute for companionship.

5. *Consider adopting or fostering a pet.* Animal companions offer lots of love, and they're also great icebreakers, as every dog walker knows. If you can't have or don't want a full-time pet, volunteer at the local animal shelter, pet-sit for friends (and grandkids), or foster pets in your home. Pet rescue organizations and those who train service animals are looking for animal lovers for short-term sheltering.

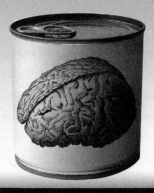

CHAPTER ELEVEN

Creativity, Spirit, and Attitude
Enrich Thyself

Not surprisingly, your emotional life affects your brain just as your brain dictates your feelings: they are inseparable. A life rich in emotional, spiritual, and intellectual experiences builds up cognitive reserve that contributes to a healthy aging brain.

Cognitive reserve is like money in the bank. The term refers to a resilience that tends to protect the brain: a set of mental skills we develop out of both our innate intelligence and attitudes and from the total of our positive and complex life experiences, especially those that are educational, emotional, and cultural. The more cognitive reserve we have, the more resilient we are and the better some people cope with life's accidents, including Alzheimer's disease.

In fact, some research suggests that engaging in leisure and creative activities makes your brain more efficient, and that cognitive reserve delays the onset and slows the progression of dementia and Alzheimer's. Backing this up is plenty of evidence that a lifestyle characterized by leisure activities of an intellectual, creative, and social nature is associated with slower cognitive decline in the healthy elderly.

It makes sense. Numerous studies have shown actual positive changes in brain structure and function in research animals who are immersed in enriched, complex environments that had a multitude of frequently changing toys and objects and other animal companions. Autopsies show increases in new dendrite branches and synapses (the areas that receive and send communication signals), and in the number of white and gray cells. These also show a cascade of molecular and neurochemical changes, such as an increase in neurotrophins— molecules that protect and grow the brain.

Cognitive reserve could help explain why some brains that are found after death to be riddled with the pathology of Alzheimer's plaques and tangles performed during life without obvious symptoms.

Just as with the rodents in so many studies whose mental performance was linked to environmental enrichment, so it is with us: cognitive reserve can tide us over many rough spots.

The Art of an Active Brain

Involvement in creative activities has long been associated with better brain health. Just look at the artists who continue producing well—and very well—into very old age. So it stands to reason that the arts can benefit nonartists as well, and a study seems to show it's true. A study sponsored by the National Endowment for the Arts begun in 2001 recruited one hundred people between the ages of 65 and 103 at three sites: the Washington, D.C., area; Brooklyn, New York; and San Francisco. The researchers divided them into two groups, with fifty participating in a weekly arts program and the others going about their usual lives. The average age of participants in all three sites was approximately 80.

The arts activities included visual arts, dance, music, poetry, drama, and oral history, all led by professional artists. After two years, those participating in the weekly art programs reported at follow-up assessments significantly better health, fewer doctor visits, less medication use, and more positive responses on the Geriatric Depression Scale and the Loneliness Scale.

Consider the power of music's good vibrations. Music not only moves the body; it sways and benefits the brain and can improve mental as well as physical well-being. Whether you turn on the Bee Gees, the Beatles, or Bach, the auditory cortex analyzes the many components of the music—volume, pitch, timbre, melody, and rhythm—and activates your brain's reward centers to depress activity in the amygdala and reduce fear and other negative emotions.

The sound of music can treat anxiety and insomnia, lower blood pressure, and soothe those with dementia. Neuroscientists recommend learning a musical instrument as a way to exercise and bolster the brain. The motor cortex, cerebellum, and corpus callosum (which connects the brain's two sides) are all bigger in musicians than in nonmusicians. And string players have more of their sensory cortices devoted to their fingers than do those who don't play the instruments. There is no agreement yet on whether musical training makes anyone smarter, but some studies have indeed shown that music lessons can improve the spatial abilities of young children.

In fact, you might say we self-medicate with music. Upbeat or exciting music boosts mood. Calming music reduces levels of the stress hormone cortisol and eases pain: think of the classic anxiety-reducing effect of a lullaby. Studies have shown music to be a powerful tool for relaxing before surgery, and gerontology researcher and nurse Linda A. Gerdner of the University of Arkansas for Medical Sciences exposed thirty-nine severely impaired Alzheimer's disease patients to music they liked twice a week for six weeks. The favored music lowered their agitation levels during and after the listening period much more than did a similar schedule of classical relaxation music they heard at a separate time.

Live Larger to Live Better

It's said that travel broadens the mind, and it might also keep it healthier. Stay-at-home seniors who spend their time restricted to their living quarters could have a higher chance of developing dementia than those who get out and about, a study suggests.

Researchers recruited almost thirteen hundred senior citizens with no signs of dementia. They had their cognitive function tested annually for up to eight years, and they also described their living space. Some, for example, mostly hung around their bedroom. Others spent time in the yard or frequently traveled.

By the end of the study, 180 people had Alzheimer's, with those whose life space narrowed in on their immediate home almost twice as likely to develop the condition as those who get up and go. The homebound folks also had an increased risk of other cognitive impairments and a faster rate of cognitive decline. "Perhaps life space is an indicator of how much we are actively engaging and challenging our cognitive abilities," says Bryan James of the Rush University Medical Center in Chicago, the study's lead investigator.

The Power of Meditation for the Aging Brain

It's hard to imagine that mere decades ago, meditation was not taken seriously by the medical profession. Numerous studies since have shown it contributes to measurable healthy physical changes in practitioners. It's a tried-and-true stress reducer, taught in stress reduction programs in thousands of hospitals and health clinics.

That's a boon for a brain growing older, because several of the conditions that meditation improves are connected with a higher risk of dementia, especially stress, depression, diabetes, and high blood pressure.

Studies are showing that meditation also acts directly on the brain. It changes the function and the physical structure of the brain in some ways specifically helpful for aging—ways that might offset some effects and risks connected with growing older and improve cognitive function.

It's a simple (but not so easy) practice, and is taught in several different forms, including Zen, Insight and Mindfulness Meditation, and transcendental meditation. Research is suggesting different meditation techniques may stimulate different parts of the brain, but all of them involve basically the same practice: sitting quietly and focusing on one sound, image, or thought and not becoming involved in other thoughts or feelings that may arise. Movement might also be part of a meditation practice.

Researchers have been illuminating the actual brain changes related to meditation through brain scans, with both practiced and novice meditators. The Dalai Lama, a supporter of science in general and neuroscience in particular, has facilitated the participation of long-time meditators, some of them monks who have been meditating for decades.

In one study, magnetic resonance imaging showed that brain regions associated with attention and sensory processing were thicker in long-time practitioners using Insight Meditation than in matched controls, and the differences were more pronounced in older participants. The suggestion is that meditation might offset age-related thinning of the prefrontal cortex and right anterior insula. Studies showed the thickness of two regions related to the length of meditation experience.

A controlled study imaged the brains of meditators and a control group before and after an eight-week trial. Those who meditated for thirty minutes using a practice called Mindfulness Meditation had measurable changes in their brains: gray matter increased in the hippocampus, important for memory and learning, and decreased in the amygdala, our internal sentry that registers fear and stress.

Another study showed increased gray matter density in the brain stem of Mindfulness meditators in areas related to cardiorespiratory activity, which could relate to the stress-relieving benefits of meditation. A study of Zen meditators showed that practitioners didn't show the gray matter volume and attention performance loss expected in relation to aging, and a University of California, Los Angeles, study found that certain regions in the brains of long-term meditators were larger than in a similar control group: the hippocampus and areas within the orbito-frontal cortex, the thalamus, and the inferior temporal gyrus, all regions known for regulating emotions. Other studies have shown that although the brain's cells typically fire at all different times, they fire in synchrony during meditation creating a stronger brain signal.

A twelve-minute Kirtan Kriya meditation technique, which involves silent and vocal chanting of four syllables while tapping fingers, resulted in positive changes in both memory and cerebral blood flow in practitioners with memory issues after eight weeks of practice.

Meditation has many pluses. It's noninvasive and low (or no) cost, and it requires thirty minutes a day or less to change your brain and possibly your mental and brain health. It has been taught for millennia in several versions in religious or spiritual practices as diverse as Judaism, Christianity, Sufism, Hinduism, Buddhism, and Zen, but it is also in wide practice among those with no interest in its spiritual aspects. It's being taught at health maintenance organizations and other health centers across the country, and one of them is probably near you.

Smile! It Could Make You Happier

You are what your face expresses, it seems. Making an emotional face—or suppressing one—influences your feelings. We smile because we are happy, and we frown because we are sad. But does the causal arrow point in the other direction too? A spate of recent studies of Botox recipients and others suggests that our emotions are reinforced, perhaps even driven, by their corresponding facial expressions.

Charles Darwin first posed the idea that emotional responses influence our feelings in 1872. "The free expression by outward signs of an emotion intensifies it," he wrote. The esteemed nineteenth-century psychologist William James went so far as to assert that a person who does not express an emotion has not felt it at all. Although few scientists would agree with such a statement today, there is evidence that emotions involve more than just the brain.

The face, in particular, appears to play a big role. When psychologist Paul Ekman, who determined that the facial expression of emotions is the same the world over, was experimenting with making faces associated with universal and powerful emotions, he found himself flooded with the emotion he was artificially expressing with his face.

So where does Botox, foe of frowning, fit into all this?

In a small study, psychologists at the University of Cardiff in Wales found that people whose ability to frown is compromised by cosmetic Botox injections are happier, on average, than people who can frown. The researchers administered an anxiety and depression questionnaire to twenty-five females, half of whom had received frown-inhibiting Botox injections. The Botox recipients reported feeling happier and less anxious in general; more important, they did not report feeling any more attractive, which suggests that the emotional effects were not driven by a psychological boost that could come from the treatment's cosmetic nature.

"It would appear that the way we feel emotions isn't just restricted to our brain—there are parts of our bodies that help and reinforce the feelings we're having," says Michael Lewis, a coauthor of the study. "It's like a feedback loop."

In a related study from the Technical University of Munich in Germany, researchers scanned Botox recipients using functional magnetic resonance imaging while asking them to mimic angry faces. They found that the Botox subjects had much lower activity in the brain circuits involved in emotional processing and responses—in the amygdala, hypothalamus, and parts of the brain stem—as compared with controls who had not received treatment.

The concept works the opposite way too, enhancing emotions rather than suppressing them. People who frown during an unpleasant procedure report feeling more pain than those who do not, according to a study published in May 2008 in the *Journal of Pain*. Researchers applied heat to the forearms of twenty-nine participants who were asked to make either unhappy, neutral, or relaxed faces during the procedure. Those who exhibited negative expressions reported being in more pain than the other two groups.

No one yet knows why our facial expressions influence our emotions. The associations in our mind between how we feel and how we react may be so strong that our expressions simply end up reinforcing our emotions; that is, there may be no evolutionary reason for the connection. Even so, our faces do seem to communicate our states of mind not only to others but also to ourselves: "I smile, so I must be happy."

Attitudes Matter: The Optimism Factor

Does attitude matter? Some studies say not. Other research says optimists not only have a cheerier outlook on life but live longer and that their brains perform better. Some studies have suggested that pessimism and fears about the losses of aging may even undermine memory and mental health, whereas optimism perks up performance.

Your brain may perform as old as your mind thinks you are—and negative expectation can be self-fulfilling. Researchers found that when older volunteers took a series of cognitive tests after being given hints that their age might affect the results, they did less well. In the study led by Thomas M. Hess of North Carolina State University, researchers worked with one hundred adults in two age groups, from 60 to 70 and from 71 to 82.

All were given a series of tasks involving arithmetic and memorization, and some of them were given the idea that test givers thought their age might affect their performance. They told them the test was being used to examine the effects of age on memory and asked the volunteers to write down their age just before taking the test.

Researchers found that those given hints that age affects performance did worse than those in the other group, especially among the young old (the 60 to 70 year olds) and those with the most education. The old old group was affected less, perhaps because they care less about being labeled.

Positive expectations had the opposite effect, as expected. A study from Wageningen University in the Netherlands interviewed 1,999 elderly Dutch men and women and found that agreement with statements such as, "I still have many goals to strive for," was highly predictive for longevity. When the same people were traced nine years after the survey, researchers found that the death rates of optimistic men were 63 percent lower than those of their pouty peers; for women, optimism reduced the rate by 35 percent.

The Dutch study also looked at other factors, such as diet, smoking, obesity, physical activity, and alcohol dependence, to try to isolate the protective influence of optimism. They found that it tends to drive healthy behavior: optimists tend to follow prescribed medical routines. A Stanford University study found also that positive attitudes are connected with longevity.

Generally those who are optimistic, agreeable, open to new experiences, conscientious, positively motivated, and goal directed are more likely to age successfully, take advantage of opportunities, cope more effectively with life circumstances, effectively regulate emotional reactions to events, and maintain a sense of well-being and life satisfaction in the face of challenge.

The opposite is also true: stress and distress, depression, anxiety, and negative emotions such as anger and shame are associated with a variety of negative outcomes, including cognitive decline. Studies have consistently found a higher level of neuroticism to be linked to an increased incidence of Alzheimer's disease and mild cognitive impairment in old age.

Fortunately, pessimists can learn to look on the bright side. Martin E. P. Seligman, a psychologist at the University of Pennsylvania not linked to the Dutch team, randomly assigned pessimistic college students to optimism workshops and found they subsequently had fewer health service visits and lower rates of depression and anxiety than classmates who had no "happiness classes."

Positive self-talk can help too, psychologists say. So perhaps we should start repeating, "Every day in every way, I'm getting better and better." What can it hurt?

PART FOUR

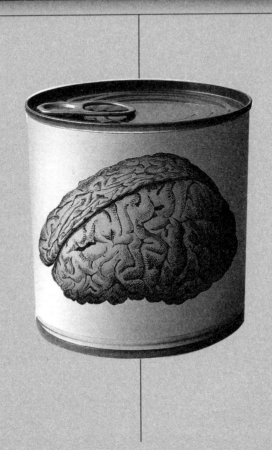

The Future for Your Brain

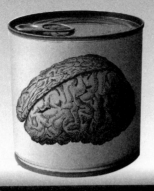

CHAPTER TWELVE

Predictions, Promises, and Possibilities

The future promises much to preserve and power our aging brains.

Just as science has produced plenty of assistive devices, spare parts, and innovative treatments to help us keep our bodies active as we age, so will our brains benefit from the amazing technology on the horizon.

Already the deaf are hearing with cochlear implants, a man paralyzed with locked-in syndrome is "speaking" through a brain electrode connected to a computerized synthesizer, and an amputee is moving a prosthetic arm by thought alone. Artificial retinas are allowing some blind to see. Deep brain implants allow a person to control Parkinson's tremors and epileptic seizures, and have been shown to ease chronic, intractable depression as well.

Some predict that within decades, we'll also be expanding our memory with microprocessor implants in our brains. Although the technologies that make bionic brain implants possible are still in an early stage, in the not-very-distant future, they may greatly expand, or fix, your brain. Neuroimplants of programmable microprocessors may turn parts of your brain into an outsized flash drive, allowing you to carry massive amounts of data and electronics inside your head, including your smart phone, your Internet access, a list of everybody's birthdays, your entire family history and contacts (including second cousins once removed), your medical history, and all your favorite books.

And this is science, not science fiction.

There's a perfect storm of events contributing to this, including unprecedented technological advances, cooperation among different sciences and even nations, and the burgeoning demands of the millions of boomers who are not going gently into that dimming of the light. Those approaching old age are clamoring for cures and aids for body and brain, and as the biggest single demographic group (and the best-off financially, even with the recession), they are pushing research forward. Billions are being expended for brain research, especially in areas related to dementia, memory loss, and other conditions of aging. The National Institutes of Health alone spent more than $13 billion, nearly 30 percent of its total budget, on overall mind- and brain-related research in 2010.

As a result of these multiple factors, researchers are making sweeping progress in both understanding and manipulating the brain. We've learned more about the brain in the past fifty years than the preceding fifty thousand, and the next two decades may even surpass that record. Brain research has moved beyond psychology, psychiatry, neurology, and even biology and married the wet and hard sciences: it now includes bioengineering, chemistry, mechanics, statistical analysis, information technologies, and even physics, with technology contributing ever better, smaller, faster, and smarter devices and techniques.

It sounds like fantasy, but scientists and futurists are predicting these aids for aging brains by midcentury:

- The brain will accept (and incorporate biologically) computer chips or mini-microprocessors to expand memory and control symptoms of brain disease from Alzheimer's to Parkinson's to depression and anxiety. And these will act as portals to receive and transmit information wirelessly: you won't need a cell phone or a computer to stay in touch.

- Brain surgery will be a thing of the past except for the most severe cases. Advanced neuroimaging will identify mental illness and brain disease before symptoms show and be in general use to "read" minds and predict and control behavior. Microscopic nanobots will enter your bloodstream to diagnose and repair disease and brain damage, rather like the 1966 film, *The Fantastic Voyage*. Protein molecules or viral vehicles will travel your brain in a similar way to turn on or off brain cells or genes responsible for brain diseases.

- Neuroenhancers, from drugs to digital devices, will boost memory and mind function in healthy and ailing brains, and equally powerful drugs will help block painful or traumatic memories. That could mean growing new brain cells to replace neurons damaged by disease—or slipping yourself a memory pill before a big event or challenge.

- Brain-machine interfaces will offer huge opportunities for the ailing aging as well as the able-bodied, such as distant control of machines and virtual touch sensations. We'll be able to run machinery, perform surgery, have virtual sex, or pilot an airplane, ocean liner, or spaceship with thought—or, more correctly, neural impulses transmitted wirelessly.

- Neurological diseases, and that includes Alzheimer's, will be preventable, curable, and even reversible in many people, as will other dementias and perhaps even mental retardation. Within a generation, some predict, nerve regeneration, or artificial nerves, could return movement to those with spinal cord injuries or debilitating nerve diseases such as multiple sclerosis and help those with Parkinson's disease.

- Both gene replacement and stem cell therapies are coming into their own, offering immense promise for curing and preventing neurological diseases. Some research has even used neural stem cells to reverse some memory loss in mice.

A Fix to Reverse Memory Decline

In the not-too-distant future, it may be possible to revive a lost ability to make memories and reverse one of the great losses of old age. Two animal studies suggest ways to approach the problem. One study connects a slowing of neurogenesis with memory loss, suggesting an avenue for possible treatment. The other involves stem cell therapy to replace damaged areas and create new networks.

Neurogenesis, the brain's ability to make new brain cells, declines as we age, and that lessened supply of new nerve cells in the adult brain may trigger short-term memory loss. Researchers from the Salk Institute for Biological Studies in La Jolla, California, confirmed this by interfering with memory formation in mice through genetic manipulation and by exposure to a cancer drug. The resulting loss in neural stem cells and memory suggests that triggering new neuron production in certain parts of older brains could stave off short-term forgetfulness, setting the stage for one day developing therapies designed to maintain a steady supply of fresh neurons to keep the mind sharp.

Another mouse experiment suggests it might be all about the networks. Frank M. LaFerla of the University of California, Irvine, and his team caused neuron death in the hippocampus by turning on specific genes. Mice whose brains were injured with this method showed significant memory impairment on place-recognition tests.

But after an injection of neural stem cells from young mice, the injured mice performed as well as healthy mice. When the researchers tracked the usual stem cells in the mouse brains, they saw that only about 5 percent of them actually developed into neurons. But mice injected with stem cells developed a far greater number of synapses at the damaged site than did the control mice.

It's a distance from these discoveries to actual therapies, but scientists are making progress that within decades could help aging brains. A major stem cell initiative is under way at the California Institute for Regenerative Medicine in San Francisco, which has $3 billion in funding from the state of California to support research at the state's universities and research institutions. The institute reports that researchers are successfully transplanting stem cells into animals with neurodegenerative diseases. In mice they've corrected the abnormal gait of Parkinson's disease, improved memory loss from an Alzheimer's disease–like condition, and eliminated the jerky body movements of Huntington's disease. The major challenges to treatment are getting enough of the right kinds of cells, getting them into the right place in the brain, and controlling the cells so they don't mutate or start a runaway process that could produce cancer.

This work gives us much to hope for. The most dreaded neurological diseases could be cured. Damage from stoke, a leading cause of death and a major crippler, could be mitigated by stem cells before the worst of the damage is done—or the damage could be prevented or fixed. Innovative therapies might fix brains damaged by many other causes, including Alzheimer's. With luck, some of these therapies now in the early stages of discovery will arrive in time to help today's senior brains.

Are You Saving for Those Final Years?

Some of these marvelous upgrades for the aging brain will no doubt be costly.

How much money do you put away each month toward your needs in those future years? Maybe you sock away all you can, already dreaming of that cruise, safari, or pied-à-terre in Paris. More realistically, you may be thinking of what aids and assists you'll need or want to make those last years comfortable, from a state-of-the-art hearing or seeing device to an electronic memory aid or full-time assistant to allow you to age in place in your very own home.

Or maybe you can't even imagine where you'll be then, what you'll want to use the money for, even what you'll be like. When you think about yourself far in the future, it's almost like thinking about someone else.

A growing body of work suggests that the more you feel your future self is really you, the more you'll put in his or her—whoops, *your*—bank account. When making decisions, we often treat our future self the way we would treat another person, found a study in 2008 by Princeton psychologist Emily Pronin. People in the study often shied away from doing something helpful but unpleasant when they had to do it right at that moment. But when their help was needed a few months or a year down the line, they were more likely to sign up—just as likely as they were to suggest that someone else should help out.

Exactly how distant we feel from our future self varies from person to person, according to a 2008 study by psychologists Hal Ersner-Hersfield and Brian Knutson, then both at Stanford University. They asked people to think about themselves now and in the future while scanning their brain with functional magnetic resonance imaging. Previous studies showed that an area of the brain called the rostral anterior cingulate cortex is activated more when you think about yourself than when you think about another person; this study showed that it is also more active when you think about yourself now as compared with imagining yourself ten years from now.

Some people showed a smaller difference in activity, suggesting they saw their future self more as "me" than as "someone else." Each participant in the study then had to pick between getting some money immediately or getting a larger sum in a certain number of days in the future. People varied in how much extra cash they required to make the reward worth the wait, and that variation, the study found, matched the brain scans: the people who showed a smaller difference in brain activity when thinking about their current and future self needed less money to make the wait worthwhile.

These individual differences affect financial decisions outside the lab too. In their next study, Ersner-Hersfield and Knutson found that people who saw their current and future self as more alike had real-world financial assets that were worth more—even when the researchers accounted for factors such as age and education. It seems the more you report feeling similar to your future self, the more savings you report having in your bank account.

RX for This Good Life

It seems that so much connected with maintaining health is uncomfortable, unpleasant, or painful, and that includes the pills, potions, needle pricks, and even surgery we need to deal with our illnesses, accidents, and chronic conditions over a lifetime.

Fortunately, the prescription for maintaining a healthy aging brain is far more pleasant. In fact, it's downright good. Research shows that your mature brain thrives on some of the very things that give pleasure and zest to life. To keep your brain at its best as you and it grow older, experts advise us to remain socially, physically, and mentally active; eat well; and be creative. And many of these overlap, yielding multiple benefits.

How fortuitous. Your brain likes socializing—spending time with friends and loved ones, just talking or playing games, dancing, making music, and cooperating on creative or community projects—and making love. Many of these fit right in with the prescription for mental exercise, especially games that require problem solving. Learning a language can be social and increase your pleasure in travel along with your brain health.

And for a happy and an active lifestyle, the findings are overwhelming in favor of the activities many of us already enjoy, such as playing sports, biking, swimming, yoga, and tai chi. Walking a mile or so a day tops the list for ease and effectiveness. Gardening can work mind and muscles and contribute to good feelings and good nutrition, along with beautifying your home and neighborhood.

Some edibles considered delicacies or sinful luxuries are major contributors to brain health—coffee, tea, dark chocolate, and the daily glass of wine—along with fresh fruit and vegetables.

You've heard about these healthy lifestyle practices, but probably in a manner that implied deprivation at worst and discipline at the very least. It's good to know that in fact, the future of your brain can be helped by practices you enjoy. What a prescription for a healthy brain!

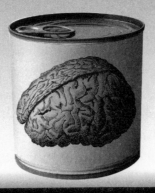

CHAPTER THIRTEEN

Living in the Now

We don't live forever, and we all know that. If we are lucky enough to live to a great old age, we'll doubtless face some disability in our final years, and of course we know that too.

Still, our brains have trouble accepting that fact, and no wonder. The vast and lucrative anti-aging industry concentrates mostly on helping us (sometimes at great expense, effort, and even pain) to forget aging and to look younger, and perhaps perform younger, than our biological age. And compared to our grandparents or even our parents, we do look, act, and perhaps feel younger as we grow old than they did at similar ages.

It's often said that our ancestors had an easier relationship with death, if only because they saw so much of it and at such young ages. This literal fact of life was the result of so many children and young adults dying prematurely. One-fourth of children died of infection before they reached the age of 5. Women died young from the complications of childbirth, men from accidents and the wounds of war, and even a young gardener, scratching his hand on a thorn, might be lost to fatal blood poisoning.

As the average life span of humans continues to lengthen (just look at the number of centenarians the world over), some scientists have begun to ponder whether this trend will continue indefinitely. Will we be able to extend our absolute life span, now apparently capped for most of us at a bit over 100? Some research suggests we may extend that limit, that drugs or changes in diet may slow metabolism or alter basic aging processes so that humans can live longer. But so far, none of the proposed longevity strategies has been proven. And so far, the facts are clear: we will, each and every one of us, die.

Most of us don't know how or when that will happen, and most of us prefer to avoid thinking about the end of our own life. Yet it's healthy to ask such questions, at least sometimes, and to resolve some issues while your brain is still in top shape, such as about who will make your health decisions and money decisions, what you want done with your stuff, and other sticky issues of mortality.

Living with an Aging Brain

There may come a time when you or your loved ones see signs of mental slippage. Your brain begins to slow down noticeably, and some day-to-day activities become more difficult.

For some of us, mild cognitive impairment and memory issues will mean we need help sorting out our finances, medications, appointments, and other activities involving planning and decisions. It can be a great relief to get help with these chores and to save our mental and physical energy for enjoying life. For some others, the time may come for full-time caregiving: the need for a companion or caregiver nearby or a health aide to help with basic living issues. Eventually that could mean moving to assisted living or a full-time care facility.

None of us likes to think about that possibility, but, then, none of us knows what the future holds. So before that should happen, now is the time to begin planning for the future and to make your wishes known. Talk to family or loved ones about the future, and about how and where you would prefer to live if you need help. If you don't have a medical power of attorney or living will, now may be the time to make one and to decide who you would like to make medical decisions if you can't any longer. In fact, this is an action most of us should take when we are still in middle age, and you may have already. This may also be the time to sort out possessions and collections and to revisit old friends and memories. You might also consider being an organ and brain donor. (See "Donate Your Brain" on the following page.)

How We (Eventually) Die

At the very end, as death takes hold, everything stops for us as we know it.

Consciousness departs. Yet at this moment, most of the body's cells are still alive. Unaware of what just happened, they carry out, to the best of their abilities, the busy business of living: the metabolic functions that support life, procuring oxygen and nutrients from the surrounding environment, and using them to generate the energy needed to make and power the activities of proteins (the main working parts of cells) and other components of our cells.

In a short while, starved of oxygen, the cells will die, and with their death, something of immense antiquity will come to its own quiet end. Every one of the cells in the body that just died—your body— could, if the records were available, trace its ancestry through an

DONATE YOUR BRAIN

One of the last gifts you might make on your way out of this life is a gift of your very own self: donations of your organs and your brain to help others and to aid research.

There's been an upsurge in donations in recent years, perhaps spurred by the recession: it changed the way many people live, and its repercussions appear to be altering how some people choose to die.

The Banner Sun Health Research Institute near Phoenix typically receives about a thousand inquiries every year about making donations. That number has increased by 15 percent since the beginning of the recession in 2008, and a waiting list for donors has lengthened.

"People have less valuation in their 401Ks, and on top of that their home values started to take a hit, so they started to look at alternative ways [of making death arrangements]," says Brian Browne, a spokesperson for the institute, which uses the donated tissue for research on Alzheimer's and Parkinson's diseases, among other disorders. Savings from forgoing cremation costs can range between a thousand and fifteen hundred dollars.

The Anatomy Gifts Registry, a nonprofit in Glen Burnie, Maryland, that supplies tissue for medical research, has seen donor calls increase from 150 to 250 a month to as many as 400, says Brent Bardsley, the registry's executive vice president, who also attributes the uptick to the downturn. Bardsley has even talked to undertakers trying to help desperate families unable to afford the full costs of a funeral. A small savings on last arrangements could translate into a valuable contribution for science and a meaningful legacy.

See the Resources section at the back of the book for information on making brain donations.

unbroken chain of cell divisions backward in time through an almost unimaginable 4 billion years to the emergence of the earliest forms of cellular life on this planet.

But some of your cells are endowed with something as near to immortality as can be attained on earth. When your death occurs, only a tiny number of your cells will continue this immortal lineage into the future—and then only if you have children. Only one cell of your body escapes extinction—a sperm or an egg—for each surviving child you produce, and as your children grow and reproduce, your cells may continue into the future.

Going Out with a Bang: The Brain Surges Just Before Death

There is no way (at least not yet) for the living to know what happens in death, but people who are resuscitated from near death often report strange sensory phenomena, such as memories flashing before their eyes or a white light or tunnel. An assessment of brain activity just before death suggests a scientific theory about such experiences.

Anesthesiologist Lakhmir Chawla of George Washington University Medical Center analyzed brain activity in seven sedated, critically ill patients as they were removed from life support and died. Electroencephalogram recordings of neural electrical activity saw a brief but significant spike at or near the time of death despite a preceding loss of blood pressure and associated drop in brain activity. The jolts lasted 30 to 180 seconds and displayed properties that are normally associated with consciousness, such as extremely fast electrical oscillations in the brain known as gamma waves. Soon after the activity abated, the patients were pronounced dead.

The event happened at what Chawla called a "very peculiar time point," when most people would think your brain would be physiologically dead because of an absence of blood flow. Chawla posits that the predeath spikes are most likely brief, "last hurrah" seizures originating in brain areas that were irritable or unstable from oxygen starvation. Living nerve cells constantly maintain an electrical charge gradient, similar to the difference in charge on the poles of a battery. Keeping up this polarity takes energy—in this case, energy created from oxygen metabolism. As blood flow slows and oxygen runs out, the cells can no longer maintain polarity and they fire, causing a cascade of activity that ripples through the brain. Chawla suggests that if these seizures were to occur in memory regions, they could explain the vivid recollections often reported by people who are resuscitated from near death, but says it's hard to speculate further because only the forebrain was monitored in this study.

The end of our individual selves has fascinated us, and religious groups from the dawn of human consciousness have speculated on the end of life and an aftermath. Science has not backed up any of the many beliefs so far.

We just don't know much about the end of life for the brain. It's a poorly researched area, and no one has come back to tell us what happens. It is, after all, the last great mystery in the life of your brain.

Living in the Now

The coming decades offer much promise for expanding knowledge and developing treatments to extend and expand our aging brains and perhaps our lifespan. Some of those amazing advances are right here, right now.

But truth be told, many reading this book may not be here to benefit from many of them. Just as our brains are benefiting from the many advances of the past, so the next generations will benefit from tomorrow's applications of today's research.

We don't know the limits yet of longevity in general, and brain longevity in particular. And while life is always uncertain, it seems a bit more so as we approach the natural end of days.

What we do know is that aging is not a disease: it's the result of living, and so far there's only one irrevocable cure for that.

Perhaps our best bet, to quote the advice of philosophers from both ancient times and the hippy sixties, is to be here now: to live the life we have been given with the brain that we have built over decades, maximizing the wondrous and all-too-short time we have in the here and now.

SOURCES

Preface

"Global Anti-Aging Products Market to Reach $291.9 Billion by 2015, According to New Report by Global Industry Analysts," WorldHealth.net, Feb. 18, 2009, http://www.worldhealth.net/news/global_anti-aging_products _market_to_rea/.

Introduction

Life expectancy statistics: Centers for Disease Control, *Health, United States, 2010*, http://www.cdc.gov/nchs/hus.htm.

What's old, anyway? Pew Research Center Social and Demographic Trends survey, "Growing Old in America: Expectations vs. Reality," 2009, http://pewresearch.org/pubs/1269/aging-survey-expectations-versus-reality. U.S. Census Bureau, "Facts for Features," 2010 Census, http://www.census.gov/newsroom/releases/archives/facts_for_features_special_editio ns/cb11-ff08 .html.

How scientists are researching your brain: Adapted from Judith Horstman, *The Scientific American Brave New Brain* (San Francisco: Jossey-Bass, 2010).

Tools for looking inside your brain: Adapted from Horstman, *The Scientific American Brave New Brain*.

Chapter One: The Well-Aged Brain

The myth of a sad old age and the major myths of aging: Scott O. Lilienfeld, Steven Jay Lynn, John Ruscio, and Barry L. Beyerstein, "Busting Big Myths,"

Scientific American Mind, Mar.–Apr. 2010. Pew Research Center Social and Demographic Trends Survey, "Growing Old in America: Expectations vs. Reality," 2009, http://pewresearch.org/pubs/1269/aging-survey-expectations -versus-reality. Marion Sonnenmoser, "Experience Versus Speed," *Scientific American Mind*, June 2005. Retirement data from Christina Bamia, Antonia Trichopoulou, and Dimitrios Trichopoulos, "Age at Retirement and Mortality in a General Population Sample: The Greek EPIC Study," *American Journal of Epidemiology*, 2008, *167*(5), 561–569.

Actually, it's getting better all the time: Scott O. Lilienfeld, Steven Jay Lynn, John Ruscio, and Barry L. Beyerstein, "Older and Sadder," from "Busting Big Myths in Popular Psychology," *Scientific American Mind*, Mar.–Apr. 2010. Katherine Harmon, "It's Getting Better All the Time," May 17, 2010, scientificamerican.com, http://www.scientificamerican.com/blog/post.cfm? id=its-getting-better-all-the-time-hap-2010-05-17. Laura Carstensen and others, "Emotional Experience Improves with Age: Evidence Based on Over Ten Years of Experience Sampling," *Psychology and Aging*, 2011, *26*, 21–33, doi:10.1037/a0021285. Arthur A. Stone and others, "A Snapshot of the Age Distribution of Psychological Well-Being in the United States," *Proceedings of the National Academy of Sciences*, June 1, 2010, pp. 9985–9990.

Great late achievers: Hampton Roy and Charles Russell, "The Encyclopedia of Aging and the Elderly," http://www.medrounds.org/encyclopedia-of-aging /2005/12/achievements-at-advanced-age-action.html. R. Coniff, "Living Longer," in E. Goldstein (ed.), *Aging* (Boca Raton, Fla.: Social Issues Resource Series, 1981).

Are grandparents safer drivers? Fred M. Henretig and others, "Grandparents Driving Grandchildren: An Evaluation of Child Passenger Safety and Injuries," *Pediatrics*, 2011, *128*, 289–295.

Do you think I'm sexy? Based on data from American Association of Retired Persons, "Sex, Romance, and Relationships: 2009 AARP Survey of Midlife and Older Adults," http://www.aarp.org/relationships/love-sex/info-05-2010/ srr_09.html. Center for Sexual Health Promotion, Indiana University, "Findings from the National Survey of Sexual Health and Behavior (NSSHB)," *Journal of Sexual Medicine*, 2010, *7*, 5, 243–373. Debra Umberson and others, "As Good as It Gets? A Life Course Perspective on Marital Quality," *Social Forces*, 2005, *84*, 493–511.

Five great things orgasm does for your aging brain: Benedetta Leuner, Erica R. Glasper, and Elizabeth Gould, "Sexual Experience Promotes Adult Neurogenesis in the Hippocampus Despite an Initial Elevation in Stress Hormones," *Public Library of Science ONE*, 2010, *5*(7), e11597, doi:10.1371/journal .pone.0011597.

A swell of centenarians: National Institute on Aging, "Unprecedented Global Aging Examined in New Census Bureau Report Commissioned by the National Institute on Aging," July 20, 2009, http://www.census.gov/newsroom/releases/archives/aging_population/cb09-108.html. Charles Q. Choi, "A Gene for Aging Smartly," *Scientific American*, Mar. 2007.

Chapter Two: How Your Brain Grows

Brain development: Adapted from John E. Dowling, *The Great Brain Debate: Nature or Nurture?* (Princeton, N.J.: Princeton University Press, 2007).

The facts about your amazing brain: Several sources, including Eric H. Chudler, "Neuroscience for Kids, Brain Facts and Figures," University of Washington, http://faculty.washington.edu/chudler/facts.html.

A brief tour of your brain: Adapted from Judith Horstman, *The Scientific American Brave New Brain* (San Francisco: Jossey-Bass, 2010).

The gray and the white: Adapted from R. Douglas Fields, "The Other Half of the Brain," *Scientific American*, Apr. 2004; "White Matter Matters," *Scientific American*, Mar. 2008. "Hidden Brain," *Scientific American Mind*, May–June 2011; and *The Other Brain* (New York: Simon & Schuster, 2009).

Too much, too young: Erica Westly, "Too Much, Too Young," *Scientific American Mind*, July–Aug. 2010.

Childhood: Michael Purdy, "Brain's Organization Switches as Children Become Adults," Washington University news release, May 14, 2009. Nico Dosenbach and others, "Prediction of Individual Brain Maturity Using fMRI," *Science*, Sept. 10, 2010, pp. 1358–1361, doi:10.1126/science.1194144.

The teen brain: Adapted from Valerie F. Reyna and Frank Farley, "Is the Teen Brain Too Rational?" *Scientific American Mind*, Dec. 2006–Jan. 2007. Leslie Sabbagh, "The Teen Brain Hard at Work," *Scientific American Mind*, Aug.–Sept. 2006.

The brain chemical and electric: Adapted from Horstman, *The Scientific American Brave New Brain*.

Get smart younger, delay dementia older: Mark Fischetti, "Delaying Dementia," *Scientific American Mind*, June 2005.

The peak years: From Horstman, *The Scientific American Brave New Brain*; Melissa Lee Phillips, "The Mind at Midlife," *Monitor on Psychology*, 2011, *42*. Jon Taylor, Quinn Kennedy, Art Noda, and Jerome Yesavage, "Pilot Age and

Expertise Predict Flight Simulator Performance: A Three-Year Longitudinal Study," *Neurology*, 2007, *68*, 648–654.

Chapter Three: Your Brain Growing Older

"Older and Sadder," from Scott O. Lilienfeld, Steven Jay Lynn, John Ruscio, and Barry L. Beyerstein, "Busting Big Myths," *Scientific American Mind*, Mar.–Apr. 2010.

The usual effects of aging: John Dowling, *The Great Brain Debate: Nature or Nurture* (Princeton, N.J.: Princeton University Press, Princeton, 2007). Jonathan Beard, "Old vs. Young," *Scientific American Mind*, Feb.–Mar. 2006. Marion Sonnenmoser, "Experience Versus Speed," *Scientific American Mind*, June 2005. Michael Falkenstein and Sascha Sommer, "Age at Work," *Scientific American Mind*, June–July 2006. "Brain Facts: A Primer on the Brain and Nervous System," Society for Neuroscience, 2003, http://www.sfn.org/index.aspx?pagename=brainfacts.

Do the brains of men and women age differently? Thomas T. Perls and Ruth C. Fretts, "Why Women Live Longer Than Men," in Women's Health: A Lifelong Guide, *Scientific American Presents*, 1998. C. Petersen and others, "Prevalence of Mild Cognitive Impairment Is Higher in Men: The Mayo Clinic Study of Aging," *Neurology*, Sept. 7, 2010, pp. 889–897.

How memory works: Adapted from R. Douglas Fields, "Making Memories Stick," *Scientific American*, Feb. 2009; "Erasing Memories," *Scientific American Mind*, Dec. 2005, and "A Pill to Remember," scientificamerican.com, Mar. 4, 2011, http://www.scientificamerican.com/blog/post.cfm?id=a-pill-to-remember-2011-03-04. Judith Horstman, *The Scientific American Brave New Brain* (San Francisco: Jossey-Bass, 2010). G. A. Carlesimo and M. Oscar-Berman, "Memory Deficits in Alzheimer's Patients: A Comprehensive Review," *Neuropsychology Review*, 1992, 3, 119–169. D. A. Fleischman and others, "Implicit Memory and Alzheimer's Disease Neuropathology," *Brain*, 2005, *128*, 2006–2015.

Why white matter matters: R. Douglas Fields, "Hidden Brain," *Scientific American Mind*," May–June 2011, and "White Matter Matters," *Scientific American*, Mar. 2008.

The aging brain: Adapted from Nikhil Swaminathan, "Partial Recall," scientificamerican.com, Dec. 5, 2007, http://www.sciam.com/article.cfm?id=partial-recall-why-memory-fades. Donald Pfaff and Nicholas D. Schiff, "The Aging

Brain: Is It Less Connected?" scientificamerican.com, Apr. 30, 2008, http://www.scientificamerican.com/article.cfm?id=the-aging-brain-is-it-les.

Forgetting may be vital to remembering: Melinda Wenner, "Forgetting to Remember," *Scientific American Mind*, Oct.–Nov. 2007.

Five things most people get wrong about memory: Adapted from Katherine Harmon, "Four Things Most People Get Wrong About Memory," scientificamerican.com, Aug. 4, 2011, http://blogs.scientificamerican.com/observations/2011/08/04/4-things-most-people-get-wrong-about-memory/. Christopher Chabris and Daniel Simons, *The Invisible Gorilla* (New York: Broadway Books, 2011), http://www.theinvisiblegorilla.com/.

The good news: Sonnenmoser, "Experience Versus Speed." Beard, "Old vs. Young." Falkenstein and Sommer, "Age at Work."

Use those words, or lose them: Nicole Branan. "Wait, Don't Tell Me," *Scientific American Mind*, Apr.–May 2008.

More easily distracted: Aimee Cunningham, "Slow to Ignore," *Scientific American Mind*, Dec. 2008–Jan. 2009, and "Memory Maintenance," *Scientific American Mind*, Sept.–Oct. 2009. Graciela Flores, "Trying to Do Too Much," *Scientific American Mind*, Sept.–Oct. 2010. Wesley C. Clapp, Michael T. Rubens, Jasdeep Sabharwal, and Adam Gazzaley, "Deficit in Switching Between Functional Brain Networks Underlies the Impact of Multitasking on Working Memory in Older Adults," *Proceedings of the National Academy of Science*, Apr. 26, 2011, pp. 7212–7217.

Chapter Four: What Can Go Wrong

Threats to your aging brain: Background and basic information from the National Institute on Aging, www.nia.nih.gov/Alzheimers/AlzheimersInformation/GeneralInfo/ and the National Institute of Neurological Disorders and Stroke, http://www.ninds.nih.gov/disorders/disorder_index.htm.

When your brain needs help: Carsten Brandenberg, "Fixing Forgetfulness," *Scientific American Mind*, Apr.–May 2006.

Signs of mental decline: Joel N. Shurkin, "Decoding Dementia," *Scientific American Mind*, Nov.–Dec. 2009.

The darkness of dementia: Background from the Alzheimer's Association, www.alz.org. Shurkin, "Decoding Dementia."

Mild cognitive impairment: "New Studies Underscore Global Importance of Mild Cognitive Impairment in Alzheimer's Disease Continuum," Alzheimer's Association International Conference, press release, July 19, 2011, http://www.alz.org/aaic/tuesday_330amCT_news_release_mci.asp. "Mild Cognitive Impairment," disease fact sheet from the UCSF Memory and Aging Center, http://memory.ucsf.edu/education/diseases/mci.

Stroke: Internet Stroke Center, "Statistics," n.d., http://www.strokecenter.org/patients/stats.html.

A healing stroke: Mark Lescroart, "The Healing Power of Touch," *Scientific American Mind*, Aug. 2011.

Knowing the signs of stroke: National Institutes of Neurological Disorders and Stroke, http://www.ninds.nih.gov/disorders/stroke/knowstroke.html#symptoms.

Parkinson's disease: National Parkinson Foundation, http://www.parkinson.org/. Konrad Schmidt and Wolfgang Oertel, "Fighting Parkinson's," *Scientific American Mind*, Feb.–Mar. 2006. Michele Solis, "Prescription: Coffee and Cigarettes," *Scientific American Mind*, Sept.–Oct. 2010. Jay L. Alberts and others, "It Is Not About the Bike, It Is About the Pedaling: Forced Exercise and Parkinson's Disease," *Exercise and Sport Sciences Reviews*, 2011, *39*(4), 177–186.

Your brain on diabetes: American Diabetes Association, http://www.diabetes.org/diabetes-basics/. Melinda Wenner, "Your Brain on Diabetes," *Scientific American*, June 2008. T. Ohara and others, "Glucose Tolerance Status and Risk of Dementia in the Community: The Hisayama Study," *Neurology*, 2011, *77*, 1126, doi:10.1212/WNL.0b013e31822f0435.

Traumatic brain injury: Steve Tokar, "Traumatic Brain Injury More Than Doubles Dementia Risk," University of California, San Francisco, news release, July 19, 2011, http://www.ucsf.edu/news/2011/07/10279/traumatic-brain-injury-more-doubles-dementia-risk. Centers for Disease Control, "Help Seniors Live Better, Longer: Prevent Brain Injury," n.d., http://www.cdc.gov/traumaticbraininjury/seniors.html.

Depression: National Institute on Aging, fact sheet, http://www.nia.nih.gov/healthinformation/publications/depression.htm. Geriatric Mental Health Foundation, fact sheet, http://www.gmhfonline.org/gmhf/consumer/factsheets/depression_factsheet.html. Hector M. Gonzalez and others, "Depression Care in the United States: Too Little for Too Few," *Archives of General Psychiatry*, 2010, *67*, 37–46. M. Tai-Seale and others, "Two-Minute Mental Health Care for Elderly Patients: Inside Primary Care Visits," *Journal of the American Geriatrics Society*, 2007, *55*, 1903–1911. Suicide information from Centers for Disease Control and Prevention, "Web-Based Injury Statistics Query and Reporting System (WISQARS)," 2010, http://www.cdc.gov/ViolencePrevention/suicide/index.html.

The legacy of cancer: Roberta Friedman, "Chemo Brain Culprit," *Scientific American Mind*, Feb.–Mar. 2008. Pascal Jean-Pierre, "Memory Impairment Common in People with a History of Cancer," news release, Third American Association for Cancer Research Conference on the Science of Cancer Health Disparities, Sept. 30–Oct. 3, 2010.

Too much of a good thing: Melinda Wenner Moyer, "It's Not Dementia, It's Your Heart Medication," *Scientific American Mind*, Sept.–Oct. 2010. "Growth in Drug Spending for the Elderly: 1992–2010," Families USA, publication no. 00-107, July 2000. Carsten Brandenberg, "Fixing Forgetfulness," *Scientific American Mind*, Apr.–May 2006. "Anticholinergic Cognitive Burden Scale," Indianapolis Discovery Network for Dementia, http://www.indydiscoverynetwork.org/AnticholienrgicCognitiveBurdenScale.html.   F. Gerretsen and B. G. Pollock, "Drugs with Anticholinergic Properties: A Current Perspective on Use and Safety," *Expert Opinion on Drug Scientific American Safety*, June 2, 2011, http://www.ncbi.nlm.nih.gov/pubmed/21635190. M. Campbell and others, "The Cognitive Impact of Anticholinergics: A Clinical Review," *Clinical Interventions in Aging*, 2009, 4, 225–233.

Your fatty brain: Moyer, "It's Not Dementia."

Chapter Five: Alzheimer's Disease

What is Alzheimer's disease? and Some facts about Alzheimer's disease: "2011 Alzheimer's Disease Facts and Figures," Alzheimer's Association, http://www.alz.org/media_media_resources.asp. Alzheimer's Disease International, "World Alzheimer Report 2011: The Global Economic Impact of Dementia," June 2011, http://www.alz.co.uk/research/world-report-2011.

Chasing the cause: Gary Stix, "Forestalling the Darkness," *Scientific American*, June 2010; Alzheimer's Disease Education and Referral Center, National Institute of Aging, http://www.nia.nih.gov/Alzheimers/ and http://www.nia.nih.gov/Alzheimers/Publications/geneticsfs.htm. Andrew Klein, "Staving Off Dementia," *Scientific American Mind*, Apr.–May 2007. Joel N. Shurkin, "Decoding Dementia," *Scientific American Mind*, Nov.–Dec. 2009. Lissy Jarvik and others, "Children of Persons with Alzheimer Disease: What Does the Future Hold?" *Alzheimer Disease and Associated Disorders*, 2008, 22, 6–20.

Connections and considerations: J. S. Sczynski and others, "Depressive Symptoms and Risk of Dementia: The Framingham Heart Study," *Neurology*, 2010, 75, 35–41. Peter Sergo, "Predicting Alzheimer's," *Scientific American Mind*, Feb.–Mar. 2008.

Anxiety and Alzheimer's disease: Nicole Branan, "Anxiety and Alzheimer's," *Scientific American Mind*, Oct.–Nov. 2007. Brian Mossop, "Strain on the Brain," *Scientific American Mind*, July–Aug. 2011. Erik B. Bloss and others, "Evidence for Reduced Experience-Dependent Dendritic Spine Plasticity in the Aging Prefrontal Cortex," *Journal of Neuroscience*, 2011, 31, 7831–7839.

Maybe its bad neural housekeeping? Vojo Deretic and Daniel J. Klionsky, "How Cells Clean House," *Scientific American*, May 2008.

The search for a cure: Stix, "Forestalling the Darkness."

Promising therapies in the works: Stix, "Forestalling the Darkness."

Looking beyond the brain: Melinda Wenner Moyer, "A Case of Low Energy," *Scientific American Mind*, Jan.–Feb. 2010. Greg Sutcliffe and others, "Peripheral Reduction of Beta-Amyloid Is Sufficient to Reduce Brain Beta-Amyloid: Implications for Alzheimer's Disease," *Journal of Neuroscience Research*, Mar. 3, 2011, doi:10.1002/jnr.22603. Marilyn Albert, Gregory Krauss, and Arnold Bakker, "Drug Improves Brain Function in Condition That Leads to Alzheimer's," *ScienceDaily*, July 20, 2011, www.sciencedaily.com/releases/2011/07/110720085822.htm. Jochen Paulus, "Lithium's Healing Power," *Scientific American Mind*, Apr.–May 2007.

An ounce of prevention: Andrew Klein, "Staving Off Dementia," *Scientific American Mind*, Apr.–May 2007. R. Douglas Fields, "Marijuana Hurts Some, Helps Others," *Scientific American Mind*, Sept.–Oct. 2009.

The Future—Without Alzheimer's: Alzheimer's Association, "2011 Alzheimer's Disease Facts and Figures," www.alz.org/downloads/Facts_Figures_2011.pdf. Alzheimer's Disease International, "World Alzheimer Report 2011," http://www.alz.co.uk/research/world-report-2011; interviews, staff, Alzheimer's Association and Alz.forum.

Chapter Six: The Big Five for Optimal Brain Function

National Institutes of Health Consensus Development Conference Statement, "Preventing Alzheimer's Disease and Cognitive Decline," NIH State-of-the-Science Conference, Apr. 26–28, 2010, http://consensus.nih.gov/2010/

alzstatement.htm. Alzheimer's Association International Conference, "New Global Model of Alzheimer's Risk Suggests a 25 Percent Reduction in Presumed Risk Factors Could Lower Alzheimer's Cases by 3 Million Worldwide," press release, July 19, 2011, http://www.alz.org/aaic/tuesday_1230amCT _news_release_riskfactors.asp. Alzheimer's Association, "2011 Alzheimer's Disease Facts and Figures," http://www.alz.org/media_media_resources.asp.

The Cognitive shop: Gary Stix, "Forestalling the Darkness," *Scientific American*, June 2010.

How to keep your brain healthy and nimble: R. C. Shah and others, "Hemoglobin Level in Older Persons and Incident Alzheimer Disease," *Neurology*, 2011, *77*, 219–226. C. Holmes and others, "Proinflammatory Cytokines, Sickness Behavior, and Alzheimer Disease," *Neurology*, 2011, *77*, 212–218. X. Song, A. Mitnitski, and K. Rockwood, "Nontraditional Risk Factors Combine to Predict Alzheimer Disease and Dementia," *Neurology*, 2011, *77*, 227–234. J. F. Dartigues and C. Féart, "Risk Factors for Alzheimer Disease: Aging Beyond Age?" *Neurology*, 2011, *77*, 206–207. "DC: Ways to Slow Brain Aging: Exercise, Estrogen, and Sleep?" *Alzheimer Research Forum News*, Nov. 18, 2011. http://www.alzforum.org/new/detail.asp?id=2970.

Chapter Seven: Exercise Your Body

Christopher Hertzog, Arthur F. Kramer, Robert S. Wilson, and Ulman Lindenberger, "Fit Body, Fit Mind?" *Scientific American Mind*, July–Aug. 2009. Christine Gorman, "The Heart-Brain Connection," *Scientific American*, Dec. 2010. "Even with Regular Exercise, People with Inactive Lifestyles More at Risk for Chronic Diseases," *ScienceDaily*, Aug. 2, 2011, http:// www.sciencedaily.com/releases/2011/08/110802091033.htm.

This brain was made for walking: Katherine Harmon, "Aerobic Exercise Bulks Up Hippocampus, Improving Memory in Older Adults," scientificamerican .com, Jan. 31, 2011, http://blogs.scientificamerican.com/observations/2011/ 01/31/aerobic-exercise-bulks-up-hippocampus-improving-memor. Kirk I. Erickson and others, "Exercise Training Increases Size of Hippocampus and Improves Memory," *Proceedings of the National Academy of Sciences*, Jan. 31, 2011, www.pnas.org/cgi/doi/10.1073/pnas.1015950108. P. Murali Doraiswamy and Benson M. Hoffman, "Can a Walk a Day Keep Alzheimer's Away?" scientificamerican.com, Nov. 25, 2008, http://www.scientificamerican.com/ article.cfm?id=fitness-and-the-brain.

It's never too late to start exercising: Hertzog, Kramer, Wilson, and Linden-berger, "Fit Body, Fit Mind?" K. I. Erickson and others, "Physical Activity Predicts Gray Matter Volume in Late Adulthood: The Cardiovascular Health Study," *Neurology*, 2010, *75*, 1415–1422. Marie-Noël Vercambre and others, "Physical Activity and Cognition in Women with Vascular Conditions," *Archives of Internal Medicine*, 2011, *171*, 1244–1250, doi:10.1001/archinternmed.2011.282.

A fine balance: Centers for Disease Control, "Falls Among Older Adults: An Overview," Sept. 16, 2011, http://www.cdc.gov/homeandrecreational/falls/adultfalls.html. Helen Lavretsky and others, "Complementary Use of Tai Chi Chih Augments Escitalopram Treatment of Geriatric Depression," *American Journal of Geriatric Psychiatry*, 2011, *19*, doi:10.1097/JGP .0b013e31820ee9e. Janice K. Kiecolt-Glaser and others, "Stress, Inflammation, and Yoga Practice," *Psychosomatic Medicine*, 2010, *72*, 113–121. Myeong Soo Lee and Edzard Ernst, "Systematic Reviews of T'ai Chi: An Overview," *British Journal of Sports Medicine*, May 16, 2011, doi:10.1136/bjsm.2010.080622. Katherine Harmon, "To Help Prevent Falls, the Elderly Should Cut Down on Meds, Increase Vitamin D, New Guidelines," scientificamerican.com, Jan. 13, 2011, http://blogs.scientificamerican.com/observations/2011/01/13/to-help-prevent-falls-the-eld-down-on-meds-increase-vitamin-d -new-guidelines-ScientificAmerican/. Cynthia Graber, "Exercising to Music Keeps Elderly Upright," scientificamerican.com, Nov. 23, 2010, http://www .scientificamerican.com/podcast/episode.cfm?id=exercising-to-music-keeps -elderly-u-10-11-23. M. E. Hackney and G. M. Earhart, "Effects of Dance on Movement Control in Parkinson's Disease: A Comparison of Argentine Tango and American Ballroom," *Journal of Rehabilitation Medicine*, 2009, *41*, 475–481.

Fear of falling cripples: Jonathan Beard, "Odd Gait," *Scientific American Mind*, Feb.–Mar. 2006.

Chapter Eight: Challenge Your Brain

Christopher Hertzog, Arthur F. Kramer, Robert S. Wilson, and Ulman Lin-denberger, "Fit Body, Fit Mind?" *Scientific American Mind*, July–Aug. 2009. Andrew Weil, *Healthy Aging* (New York: Knopf, 2005). Kaspar Mossman, "Brain Trainers," *Scientific American Mind*, Apr.–June 2009, and "Driving and the Brain," *Scientific American Mind*, Jan.–Feb. 2010.

Educated brains stay better longer: Catherine M. Roe and others, "Alzheimer Disease and Cognitive Reserve: Variation of Education Effect with Carbon 11–Labeled Pittsburgh Compound B Uptake," *Archives of Neurology*, 2008, *65*, 1467–1471. Ellen Bialystok and others, "Bilingualism, Aging, and Cognitive Control: Evidence from the Simon Task," *Psychology and Aging*, 2004, *19*, 290–303.

Why testing boosts learning: Andrea Anderson, "Why Testing Boosts Learning," *Scientific American Mind*, Jan.–Feb. 2010.

Do brain fitness products work? Robert Goodier, "Brain Training's Unproven Hype," *Scientific American Mind*, July–Aug. 2009. P. Murali Doraiswamy and Marc E. Agronin, "Brain Games: Do They Really Work?" scientificamerican.com, Apr. 28, 2009, http://www.scientificamerican.com/article.cfm?id=brain-games-do-they-really. Mossman, "Brain Trainers." Anya Martin, "Brain Fitness Industry Set to Boom," *Marketwatch*, May 18, 2009, http://articles.moneycentral.msn.com/Insurance/InsureYourHealth/brain-fitness-industry-set-to-boom.aspx.

Computer training may keep you driving longer: Mossman, "Driving and the Brain."

The bottom line: P. Doraiswamy and Agronin, "Brain Games."

Chapter Nine: Nutrition

Ingrid Kiefer, "Brain Food," *Scientific American Mind*, Oct.–Nov. 2007. Mary Franz, "Your Brain on Blueberries." *Scientific American Mind*, Jan.–Feb. 2011. Rachel A. Whitmer and others, "Obesity in Middle Age and Future Risk of Dementia: A 27 Year Longitudinal Population Based Study," *British Medical Journal*, 2005, *330*(7504), 1360, doi:10.1136/bmj.38446.466238.E0. P. H. Chaves and others, "Association Between Mild Anemia and Executive Function Impairment in Community-Dwelling Older Women: The Women's Health and Aging Study II," *Journal of the American Geriatric Society*, 2006, *54*, 1429–1435. Lucy Wilkinson, A. B. Scholey, and K. Wesnes, "Chewing Gum Selectively Improves Memory in Healthy Volunteers," *Appetite*, 2002, *38*, 235–236.

Provisions for brain power: "Brain Food," *Scientific American Mind*, Oct.–Nov. 2007.

Glucose is not so sweet to the brain: Nikhil Swaminathan, "An End to Senior Moments," *Scientific American Mind*, Apr.–May 2009.

Forget the fructose: Aimee Cunningham, "Forget the Fructose," *Scientific American Mind*, July–Aug. 2009.

Omega-3, the essential oil: J. K. Kiecolt-Glaser and others, "Omega-3 Supplementation Lowers Inflammation and Anxiety in Medical Students: A Randomized Controlled Trial," *Brain, Behavior, and Immunity*, 2011, 25, 1725–1734. W. S. Lim and others, "Omega 3 Fatty Acid for the Prevention of Dementia," *Cochrane Database of Systematic Reviews*, 2006, art. CD005379, doi:10.1002/14651858.CD005379.pub2. C. Samieri and others, "Olive Oil Consumption, Plasma Oleic Acid, and Stroke Incidence: The Three-City Study," *Neurology*, June 15, 2011, doi:10.1212/WNL.0b013e318220abeb.

Your brain on berries, chocolate, and wine: Franz, "Your Brain on Blueberries." Kiefer, "Brain Food." Midori Natsume and others, "Cacao Polyphenols Influence the Regulation of Apolipoprotein in HepG2 and Caco2 Cells," *Journal of Agricultural and Food Chemistry*, 2011, 59, 1470–1476.

Flavors of flavonoids: Franz, "Your Brain on Blueberries."

A tipple a day is good for your brain: Edward J. Neafsey and Michael A. Collins, "Moderate Alcohol Consumption and Cognitive Risk," *Neuropsychiatric Disease Treatment*, 2011, 7, 465–484, doi:10.2147/NDT.S23159. Jim Ritter, "Moderate Social Drinking Helps Protect Against Dementia and Cognitive Impairment," Loyola University Medicine news release, Aug. 11, 2011.

Antioxidants might slow hearing loss: Sandy Fritz, "Preventing Hearing Loss," *Scientific American Mind*, May–June 2010.

Caffeine: Dwayne Godwin and Jorge Cham, "How Much Is Too Much Coffee?" *Scientific American Mind*, Jan.–Feb. 2010. Susan Cosier, "Coffee Breakdown," *Scientific American Mind*, July–Aug. 2009.

Is there a pill for that? Katherine Harmon, "Gingko Doesn't Slow Cognitive Decline in Elderly," scientificamerican.com, Dec. 29, 2009, http://www.scientificamerican.com/article.cfm?id=gingko-doesnt-slow-cognit. Gary Stix, "Spice Healer," scientificamerican.com, Jan. 14, 2007, http://www.scientificamerican.com/article.cfm?id=spice-healer. G. M. Cole, B. Teter, and S. A. Frautschy, "Neuroprotective Effects of Curcumin," *Advances in Experimental Medical Biology*, 2007, 595, 197–121. A. D. Smith and others, "Homocysteine-Lowering by B Vitamins Slows the Rate of Accelerated Brain Atrophy in Mild Cognitive Impairment: A Randomized Controlled Trial," *Public Library of Science ONE*, 2010, 5, e12244, doi:10.1371/journal.pone.0012244. Gale Smith, "B-Complex Vitamins May Help Slow

Progression of Dementia," Methodist Hospital, Houston, news release, Oct. 25, 2010, http://www.methodisthealth.com/body.cfm?id=495&action=detail&ref=719. Diane Welland, "Does D Make a Difference?" *Scientific American Mind*, Nov.–Dec. 2009. Luz E. Tavera-Mendoza and John H. White, "Cell Defenses and the Sunshine Vitamin," *Scientific American*, Nov. 2007. Katherine Harmon, "To Help Prevent Falls, the Elderly Should Cut Down on Meds, Increase Vitamin D: New Guidelines," scientificamerican.com, Jan. 13, 2011.

Chapter Ten: The Social Treatment

Katherine Harmon, "Social Ties Boost Survival by 50 Percent," scientificamerican.com, July 28, 2010, http://www.scientificamerican.com/article.cfm?id=relationships-boost-survival. Julianne Holt-Lunstad, Timothy B. Smith, and J. Bradley Layton, "Social Relationships and Mortality Risk: A Meta-Analytic," *Proceedings of the Library of Science Medicine*, 2010, 7(7), e1000316, doi:10.1371/journal.pmed.1000316. Karen A. Ertel, M. Maria Glymour, and Lisa F. Berkman, "Effects of Social Integration on Preserving Memory Function in a Nationally Representative U.S. Elderly Population," *American Journal of Public Health*, 2008, *98*, 1215–1220. Valerie C. Crooks and others, "Social Network, Cognitive Function, and Dementia Incidence Among Elderly Women," *American Journal of Public Health*, 2008, *98*, 1221–1227. Bryan D. James, Robert S. Wilson, Lisa L. Barnes, and David A. Bennett, "Late-Life Social Activity and Cognitive Decline in Old Age," *Journal of the International Neuropsychological Society*, 2011, *17*, 998–1005, doi:10.1017/S1355617711000531.

You've got a friend, we hope: Harmon, "Social Ties Boost Survival by 50 Percent." Victoria Stern, "So Lonely It Hurts," *Scientific American Mind*, May–June 2008. John T. Cacioppo and others, "In the Eye of the Beholder: Individual Differences in Perceived Social Isolation Predict Regional Brain Activation to Social Stimuli," *Journal of Cognitive Neuroscience*, 2009, *21*, 83–92, doi:10.1162/jocn.2009.21007. Klaus Manhart, "Good Friends," *Scientific American Mind*, Apr.–June 2006.

Talk to teens, live longer: Erica Westly, "Talk to Teens Live Longer," *Scientific American Mind*, Aug.–Sept. 2008.

Five great things socializing does for your brain: Judith Horstman, *The Scientific American Book of Love, Sex, and the Brain* (San Francisco: Jossey-Bass, 2011).

Finding and making friends in later life: Adapted from Horstman, *The Scientific American Book of Love, Sex, and the Brain*.

Chapter Eleven: Creativity, Spirit, and Attitude

The art of an active brain: Gene D. Cohen, "The Creativity and Aging Study: The Impact of Professionally Conducted Cultural Programs on Older Adults," National Center for Creative Aging, Apr. 2006, www.nea.gov/resources/accessibility/CnA-Rep4-30-06.pdf. Emily Anthes, "Six Ways to Boost Brain Power," *Scientific American Mind*, Feb.–Mar. 2009.

Live larger to live better: Bryan James and others, "Life Space and Risk of Alzheimer Disease, Mild Cognitive Impairment, and Cognitive Decline in Old Age," *American Journal of Geriatric Psychiatry*, 2011, *19*, 961–969.

The power of meditation for the aging brain: Anthes, "Six Ways to Boost Brain Power." Robert Schneider and others, "Effects of Stress Reduction on Clinical Events in African Americans with Coronary Heart Disease: A Randomized Controlled Trial," *Circulation*, 2009, *120*, S461. Britta Hölzel and others, "Mindfulness Practice Leads to Increases in Regional Brain Gray Matter Density," *Psychiatry Research: Neuroimaging*, 2011, *191*, 36–43. Heleen A. Slagter and colleagues, "Mental Training Affects Distribution of Limited Brain Resources," *Proceedings of the Library of Science Biology*, 5(6), e138. doi:10.1371/journal.pbio.0050138.

Smile! Melinda Wenner, "Smile! It Could Make You Happier," *Scientific American Mind*, Sept.–Oct. 2009.

Attitudes matter: Thomas M. Hess, Joey T. Hinson, and Elizabeth A. Hodges, "Moderators of and Mechanisms Underlying Stereotype Threat Effects on Older Adults' Memory Performance," *Experimental Aging Research*, 2009, *35*, 153–177, doi:10.1080/036107308027164132009. Lisa DeKeukelaere, "Optimism Prolongs Life," *Scientific American Mind*, Feb.–Mar. 2006.

Chapter Twelve: Predictions, Promises, and Possibilities

Judith Horstman, *The Scientific American Brave New Brain* (San Francisco: Jossey-Bass, 2010). U.S. Department of Health and Human Services, National Institutes of Health, "Estimates of Funding for Various Research, Condition, and Disease Categories (RCDC)," Feb. 14, 2011, http://report.nih.gov/rcdc/categories/.

A fix to reverse memory decline: Nicole Branan, "Stem Cells for Memory," *Scientific American Mind*, Feb.–Mar. 2008. Nikhil Swaminathan, "Is Old Age Memory Decline Reversible?" scientificamerican.com, Jan. 31, 2008, http://www.scientificamerican.com/article.cfm?id=is-old-age-memory-decline-reversible.

Are you saving for those final years? Valerie Ross, "When I'm 64," *Scientific American Mind*, July–Aug. 2010.

Chapter Thirteen: Living in the Now

Thomas Kirkwood, "Why We Can't Live Forever," *Scientific American*, Sept. 2010.

Donate your brain: Gary Stix, "Donate Your Brain, Save a Buck," *Scientific American*, Jan. 2011.

Going out with a bang: Peter Sergo, "Going Out with a Bang," *Scientific American Mind*, May–June 2010.

ILLUSTRATION CREDITS

Some of Your Brain's Most Important Parts: Courtesy Alzheimer's Disease Education and Referral Center, a service of the National Institute on Aging.

Why Can't We Live Forever? From Thomas Kirkwood, "Why Can't We Live Forever?" *Scientific American*, Sept. 2010. Artist: Jason Lee.

How the Brain Makes New Neurons: From Fred H. Gage, "Brain, Repair Yourself," *Scientific American*, Sept. 2003. Artist: Alice Chen.

How Learning Helps Save Neurons: From Tracy J. Shors, "Saving New Brain Cells," *Scientific American*, Mar. 2009. Artist: Jen Christiansen.

How Myelin Is Made: From R. Douglas Fields, "White Matter Matters," *Scientific American*, Mar. 2008. Artist (main image): Alan Hoofring/ NIH Med Art; Artist (insert): Jen Christiansen.

Glial Cells and Neurons: A Working Partnership: From R. Douglas Fields, "The Other Half of the Brain," *Scientific American*, Apr. 2004. Artist: Jeff Johnson/Hybrid Medical Animation.

Less Is More in Brain Development: Courtesy Dr. Paul M. Thompson, Laboratory of Neuro Imaging at UCLA.

Stroke: The Brain Attack: Courtesy National Heart, Lung, and Blood Institute, National Institutes of Health, U.S. Department of Health and Human Services.

Parkinson's Disease: Losing Motor Control: From Konrad Schmidt and Wolfgang Oertel, "Fighting Parkinson's," *Scientific American Mind*, Feb.–Mar. 2006. Artist: Sara Chen.

When the Cleaning Stops: From Vojo Deretic and Daniel J. Klionsky, "How Cells Clean House," *Scientific American*, May 2008. Artist: Jen Christiansen.

Brain Shrinkage in Alzheimer's Disease: From Gary Stix, "Forestalling the Darkness," *Scientific American*, June 2010. Artist: Andrew Swift Illustrations.

New Tools Detect Silent Early Signs of Dementia: From Gary Stix, "Forestalling the Darkness," *Scientific American*, June 2010. Artist: Andrew Swift Illustrations.

How Exercise Helps Your Brain Health: Courtesy Dr. Cyrus A. Raji/ Radiological Society of North America.

GLOSSARY

acetylcholine—a neurotransmitter that appears to regulate memory and controls muscle action in the peripheral nervous system. Alzheimer's disease is associated with a shortage of acetylcholine.

addiction—an uncontrollable craving for drugs, alcohol, or some behaviors despite adverse health, social, or legal consequences.

adrenaline—a hormone and neurotransmitter that boots up the body to participate in the fight-or-flight response of the sympathetic nervous system. Also known as epinephrine.

allele—describes one of two or more versions of a gene. *See* apolipoprotein E (ApoE) gene.

Alzheimer's disease—a type of dementia; a progressive, neurodegenerative disease caused by cell death in several areas of the brain.

amygdala—an almond-shaped area deep in the midbrain. Part of the limbic system (sometimes called the "emotional brain"), it's the survival-oriented brain part that regulates primitive emotions and the fight-or-flight syndrome.

anterior cingulate cortex—the brain area that regulates emotional states and helps people control their impulses and monitor their behavior for mistakes.

anticholinergic agents—medications that interfere with the function of acetylcholine, a neurotransmitter essential for good brain function.

antioxidants—chemical compounds found in many foods that protect cells from damage caused by free radicals. Flavonoids, polyphenolics, and the vitamins C and E are examples,

SOURCE: This information was compiled from several sources, including the National Institutes of Health.

apolipoprotein E (ApoE) gene—a gene on chromosome 19 involved in making a protein that helps carry cholesterol and other types of fat in the bloodstream. It comes in several forms, or alleles: the ApoE4 form is considered a risk-factor gene for Alzheimer's disease.

autism—a complex neurodevelopmental disorder that typically appears before age 3 and affects social interaction and communication skills.

autophagy—a process by which the body cleans up and digests damaged and dying cells, aberrant proteins, and other by-products of metabolism in the cytoplasm inside cells.

axon—the long extension from a neuron that transmits outgoing signals to other cells.

beta-amyloid—a protein fragment present at low levels in healthy brains but can accumulate to toxic levels as in Alzheimer's disease, where it forms plaques between brain cells.

biomarker—a laboratory measurement of a biological process in human tissues, cells, or fluids. These may reflect the presence or activity of a disease process or perhaps predict disease.

brain-derived neurotrophic factor (BDNF)—a growth factor synthesized in the brain that stimulates neurite outgrowth and supports survival of neurons.

brain stem—the most primitive brain part; takes care of the automated basics, such as breathing, heart beat, digestion, reflexive actions, sleeping, and arousal.

cannabinoids—compounds naturally produced in the body that have a structure similar to the psychoactive compounds found in cannabis (marijuana) and that serve as signaling molecules in the brain; endogenous cannabinoids.

caudate nucleus—located near the center of the brain on the thalamus; important in learning and memory and is intimately connected to dopamine. *See also* dopamine.

centenarian—a person who is or lives beyond the age of 100 years. Some call those past the age of 100 "supercentenarians."

cerebellum—two peach-size mounds of folded brain tissue located at the top of the brain stem that control skilled, coordinated movement (such as returning a tennis serve) and are involved in some learning pathways.

cerebral cortex—the outer three millimeters of gray matter that consist of closely packed neurons that control most body functions, including the mysterious state of consciousness, the senses, the body's motor skills, reasoning, and language. Also referred to as the neocortex.

cerebrum—the "thinking brain"; accounts for about two-thirds of the brain's mass and is positioned over and around most other brain structures. It's divided into two hemispheres (*see* corpus callosum) and four lobes, and is crowned by the cerebral cortex.

chemo brain—term for memory and concentration problems associated with chemotherapy, radiation, and other cancer treatments.

cholesterol—a waxy substance that provides structure to the body's cell membranes and is important in the brain for forming neuronal connections; in large amounts, contributes to artery damage and heart disease.

chromosome—a compact structure containing DNA and proteins present in nearly all cells of the body. Chromosomes carry genes, which direct the cell to make proteins and direct a cell's construction, operation, and repair. Normally each cell has forty-six chromosomes in twenty-three pairs. Each biological parent contributes one of each pair of chromosomes.

cognitive reserve—an unconscious mental resilience we develop out of both our innate intelligence and attitudes and from the totality of our positive and complex life experiences, especially educational, emotional, and cultural experiences. Such reserve is believed to help brains retain cognitive function even after damage or disease.

computed axial tomography imaging (CAT)—a brain imaging technique that uses X-rays and computers to show body sections behind other parts and in much more detail. Also referred to as computed tomography (CT).

corpus callosum—a band of nerve tissue that connects the two halves (or hemispheres) of the brain.

cortex—Latin for "bark," it refers to the outermost layer of the brain.

corticosterone—a glucocorticoid; a steroid produced naturally in the body that protects against stress.

cortisol—a glucocorticoid; an important steroid neurohormone that contributes to alertness and is produced in response to stress; related to corticosterone.

deep brain stimulation (DBS)—the delivery of low-level electrical stimulation via electrodes implanted in specific brain areas to block brain signals contributing to seizures, tremors, and other conditions.

dementia—the decline of short-term memory and thinking due to damage to brain cells and neural networks from a number of causes, including Alzheimer's disease.

dementia with Lewy bodies—the second most common type of dementia, in which abnormal structures develop in parts of the brain.

dendrite—an extension of the neuron that receives information from other brain cells.

dentate gyrus—one of two sections in the hippocampus; an area that generates new neurons.

diabetes—a serious progressive disease caused by an inability to produce insulin (type 1) or to process insulin (type 2).

diffusion tensor imaging (DTI)—a brain imaging technique that measures the flow of water molecules along the white matter, or myelin, of the brain, which connects many regions.

DNA—the deoxyribonucleic acid inherited from ancestors; it makes up each person's genome (or genetics) and contains the instructions for making his or her unique body and brain.

dopamine—a neurotransmitter vital for voluntary movement, attentiveness, motivation, and pleasure. It's a key player in the reward circuit and addiction, and its lack is a cause of Parkinson's disease.

electroencephalography (EEG)—a method of detecting and recording brain activity from electrodes placed on the scalp.

endorphins—naturally occurring neurohormones that reduce pain sensations and increase pleasure. The name comes from end(ogenous) (m)orphine.

epigenetics—the study of how gene expression is affected by the environment without changing the underlying coding of DNA. Also called the epi(above) genome.

epigenome—*see* epigenetics.

epinephrine—a neurotransmitter that keeps us alert and is produced and released by the adrenal glands in times of stress. Too much can increase anxiety or tension. Also called adrenaline.

erectile dysfunction, (ED)—in men, an inability to get or sustain an erection.

estrogen—a steroid hormone that makes women female, regulates reproductive cycles and menstruation, and is important for mental health. Men need some estrogen for sperm production and, possibly, desire.

executive function—mental processes that help connect past experience with present action. People use it to perform activities such as planning, organizing, strategizing, paying attention to and remembering details, and managing time and space.

familial Alzheimer's disease—also called early-onset Alzheimer's disease. A genetic condition in perhaps 1 percent of people that invariably leads to the disease, usually before age 60 and sometimes before age 40.

flavonoids—chemical compounds in many foods that act as antioxidants to protect cells from damage caused by unstable molecules known as free radicals.

free radicals—the rogue chemicals formed by our own bodies during metabolism (and also spawned by pollution, cigarette smoke, and radiation) that cause cell damage.

frontal lobes—the most recently evolved part of the brain and the last to develop in young adulthood; contains the brain's top executive and is responsible for so-called higher functions, including thinking, planning, and verbal skills.

fructose—a substance that comes from many plants, including sugarcane, sugar beets, and corn. High fructose corn syrup is used to sweeten many processed foods. Also called fruit sugar.

functional magnetic resonance imaging (fMRI)—a type of brain scan that can be used to monitor the brain's activity and detect abnormalities in how it works.

fusiform gyrus—section in the temporal lobes that is involved in recognizing faces, bodies, numbers, and words.

GABA (gamma-aminobutyric acid)—a neurotransmitter produced by neurons that slows everything down and helps keep your system in balance. It helps regulate anxiety.

gene—a segment of DNA found on a chromosome that acts as a blueprint for making virtually every biomedical reaction and structure in the body.

genome—the sum of all the genes that code for a particular organism, such as your body and brain.

glia, glial cells—the cells of the brain and nervous system that support and protect neurons and form the myelin that insulates nerve cells and improves transmission of nerve signals.

glucocorticoids—steroid hormones that play a central role in the stress response and are also involved in the metabolism of the sugar glucose and maintenance of normal glucose concentrations in the blood, have anti-inflammatory effects, and can help suppress the immune response.

glucose—a major source of energy for most cells, including those in the brain, which operate best when blood glucose levels are stable.

glutamate—a major excitatory neurotransmitter, dispersed widely throughout the brain; involved in learning and memory.

hemorrhagic stroke—a stroke caused by a bleed in the brain; usually caused by broken blood vessels.

hippocampus—a structure located deep within the brain that plays a major role in learning and memory and is involved in converting short-term to long-term memory.

homocysteine—an amino acid in the blood.

hyperglycemia—very high levels of blood glucose such as with diabetes. Can lead to damage to nerves, blood vessels, and other body organs and may cause loss of consciousness.

hypoglycemia—very low levels of blood sugar, which can starve the brain of energy, causing headache, mild confusion, abnormal behavior, loss of consciousness, seizure, and coma.

hypothalamus—a structure in the brain under the thalamus that monitors activities such as body temperature and food intake, blood pressure, and other body functions, and sets off the chemical reaction to fight or flee.

immunotherapy—treatment to stimulate or restore the ability of the immune system to fight infection and disease. One of the most promising treatments for Alzheimer's disease involves vaccines to trigger the body's immune system to produce antibodies to attack beta-amyloid.

insula—a part of the cortex active in synthesizing information, self-awareness, cognitive functioning, and interpersonal experience.

ischemic stroke—a stroke caused by a blood clot; the most common type of stroke.

levodopa (L-dopa)—a medication for Parkinson's disease that is converted to dopamine in the brain, replacing the neurotransmitter lost to disease.

limbic system—brain areas that link the brain stem with the higher reasoning elements of the cerebral cortex; sometimes called the emotional brain because it controls emotions, instinctive behavior, and the sense of smell.

magnetic resonance imaging (MRI)—a computer image of internal structures in the body generated by magnetic fields. This technique is particularly good for imaging the brain and soft tissues.

magnetoencephalography (MEG)—measures the magnetic fields created by electric current flowing within neurons and detects brain activity associated with various functions in real time.

metabolism—all of the chemical processes that take place inside the body.

mild cognitive impairment (MCI)—a loss of cognitive function that doesn't always progress to dementia, doesn't include personality changes, and isn't always due to Alzheimer's disease.

mitochondria—the cellular component that's responsible for energy production in cells.

myelin—a whitish, fatty insulating layer surrounding an axon that helps the axon rapidly transmit electrical messages from the cell body to the synapse. Also called white matter or referred to as a myelin sheath.

neocortex—*see* cerebral cortex.

neural—anything related to neurons, which are brain cells.

neurite—an outgrowth from a nerve cell that can be an axon or a dendrite.

neurofibrillary tangles—damaging formations inside brain cells caused by abnormal tau protein and one of the hallmarks connected with Alzheimer's disease.

neurogenesis—the ability of the brain to generate new cells, or neurons, in certain areas.

neuron—a nerve or brain cell.

neuroplasticity—the brain's ability to change in response to the environment, including thoughts and feelings, and to reassign some of its parts to take over new tasks.

neurotransmitter—a chemical messenger between neurons, released by the axon on one neuron to excite or inhibit activity in a neighboring neuron; sometimes a hormone.

nucleus accumbens—part of the brain's reward system, located in the limbic system, that processes information related to motivation and reward. Intimately involved in sexual arousal and drug addiction.

occipital lobe—processes and routes visual data to other parts of the brain for identification and storage.

omega-3 fatty acid—found in coldwater fish and flax seed, it contributes to heart, brain, and joint health; available in fish oil and flax supplements, the eggs of specially fed chickens, and added to some foods.

oxytocin—a neurohormone produced in the brains of newborns, nursing mothers, and at orgasm. It's the hormone of love, trust, and attachment and is involved in bonding.

parietal lobes—one of the four subdivisions of the cerebral cortex, they receive and process sensory information from the body, including language, and are involved in attention.

Parkinson's disease—a progressive neurological disease due to a gradual degeneration of the brain cells that produce dopamine, the neurotransmitter that helps control voluntary movement.

plasticity—the ability of the brain to change through the formation or strengthening of connections between neurons in the brain. See neuroplasticity.

polyphenolics—a class of antioxidants found in many foods, including berries such as acai and strawberries and grapes and red wine.

positron emission tomography (PET)—an imaging technique using radioisotopes that allows researchers to observe and measure activity in different parts of the brain by monitoring blood flow and concentrations of substances such as oxygen and glucose, as well as other specific constituents of brain tissues.

prefrontal cortex—the brain region involved in planning complex cognitive behaviors, personality expression, decision making, and moderating correct social behavior.

protein—a substance that determines the physical and chemical characteristics of a cell and therefore of an organism. Proteins are essential to all cell functions and are created using genetic information.

senile plaques—large accumulations of the toxic protein beta-amyloid in the brains of people with Alzheimer's disease; also to a smaller amount with healthy aging.

serotonin—a neurotransmitter that helps regulate body temperature, memory, emotion, sleep, appetite, and mood.

single photon emission computed tomography (SPECT)—a brain imaging technique that uses a small amount of radioactive tracer to measure and monitor blood flow in the brain and produce a three-dimensional image.

social networks—any kind of network of acquaintances and friends, but used today to apply to virtual or Internet services and connections such as Facebook.

statins—a class of cholesterol-lowering drugs.

stem cells—cells with the ability to divide for indefinite periods and to give rise to specialized cells. They are the subject of intense research and controversy, since embryos provide a source of undifferentiated stem cells.

stroke—an interruption of blood flow to the brain resulting in the death of brain cells due to lack of oxygen; caused by a blockage (ischemic) or a bleed (hemorrhagic) incident.

synapse—the tiny gap between neurons across which chemicals such as neurotransmitters pass, and by which cells share information.

tau—a protein important in transporting nutrients in the brain. In Alzheimer's disease, abnormal tau forms, damaging neurofibrillary tangles inside brain cells.

temporal lobes—brain area that controls the memory storage area and hears and interprets music, language, and emotion. When stimulated, may produce feelings of spirituality.

tetrahydrocannabinol (THC)—the active ingredient in marijuana that gives it hallucinogenic properties.

thalamus—located at the top of the brain stem. Acts as a two-way relay station, sorting, processing, and directing signals from the spinal cord and midbrain structures up to the cerebrum, and, conversely, from the cerebrum down the spinal cord to the nervous system.

tissue plasminogen activator (tPA)—a medication that can dissolve blood clots; given in the early hours after an ischemic stroke, can often lessen disability.

transient ischemic attacks (TIAs)—a series of small ischemic strokes over time that briefly block blood flow to the brain and can cause cumulative damage.

traumatic brain injury (TBI)—a brain injury that can lead to cognitive problems.

U.S. Food and Drug Administration (FDA)—the federal agency that regulates pharmaceutical products and medical devices.

vascular dementia—the second most common type of dementia, typically (but not always) a series of symptoms following a stroke.

ventral tegmental area (VTA)—located in the midbrain at the top of the brain stem, the VTA is one of the most primitive parts of the brain. It synthesizes dopamine, which is sent to the nucleus accumbens.

white matter—myelin made up of glial cells; accounts for about half of the brain and is essential for efficient and effective communication among the 100 billion neurons in every person.

working memory—the ability to hold information in your mind for a usually brief period, such as when transferring a phone number from your address book to your smart phone or when holding or following a conversation.

The following organizations provide reliable information related to many aspects of aging. Your doctor can help you find local resources.

Organizations on Aging

Administration on Aging, Department of Health and Human Services. A comprehensive source for information on many services for seniors, including federal and other programs and benefits, elder care, home care, health and disease information, and elder rights. htpp://www .aoa.gov/

American Geriatrics Society, Foundation for Health in Aging. Founded by the American Geriatrics Association to provide information on research and special issues related to health and aging. http://www .healthinaging.org

Eldercare Locator (Administration on Aging). A public service of the U.S. Administration on Aging connecting you to services for older adults and their families. 1-800-677-1116; www.eldercare.gov

Family Caregiver Alliance. An organization providing support services for those struggling to provide long-term care for a loved one and to help caregivers locate support services in their communities. www .caregiver.org

Geriatric Mental Health Foundation. Established by the American Association for Geriatric Psychiatry to raise awareness of psychiatric issues of the aging and to provide information. http://www .gmhfonline.org/gmhf/

National Institute on Aging. One of the twenty-seven institutes and centers of the National Institutes of Health, it leads a broad scientific effort to understand the nature of aging and to extend the healthy, active years of life. It's the primary federal agency on Alzheimer's disease research. www.nia.nih.gov/

For Alzheimer's Disease and Other Neurological Conditions

Alzheimer Research Forum. A Web site dedicated to scientific research, conference news, and news of clinical trials. http://www.alzforum.org/

Alzheimer's Association. A global voluntary health organization in Alzheimer's care, research, and support; the largest private, nonprofit funder of Alzheimer's research. http://www.alz.org/index.asp

Alzheimer's Disease Education and Referral (ADEAR). The National Institute on Aging Alzheimer's disease Web site. www.nia.nih.gov/ alzheimers

Alzheimer's Disease Research. A program of the American Health Assistance Foundation. http://www.ahaf.org/alzheimers/

American Diabetes Association. www.diabetes.org/

American Health Assistance Foundation. An international nonprofit organization funding research and providing information and coping strategies on age-related degenerative diseases including Alzheimer's disease, macular degeneration, and glaucoma. http://www.ahaf.org/

Brain Injury Association of America. http://www.biausa.org/

Living with Parkinson's: The Michael J. Fox Foundation for Parkinson's Research. www.michaeljfox.org/living.cfm

National Institute of Neurological Disorders and Stroke. www.ninds.nih.gov

National Parkinson Foundation. http://www.parkinson.org/

National Stroke Association. www.stroke.org/

Volunteer or Donate for Research

Many organizations and research centers seek volunteers, both healthy persons and those who have a neurological disease, to participate in studies. Some researchers also need tissue, blood, and brain samples for research. Healthy organs for transplant are in short supply, and age is not a barrier.

Alzheimer's Forum. Maintains a list of projects seeking participants of many kinds for research related to Alzheimer's. http://www.alzforum.org/bboards/forum_topics.asp?FID=4

Boston University Alzheimer's Disease Center. One of many centers that seeks donation of brain tissue after death for research. A brochure can be downloaded from the site. http://www.bu.edu/alzresearch/research/memory/hope/brain.html

Brain banks. For donating a brain or tissue for research. An international and national list of sites that perform postmortem diagnosis of Alzheimer's disease and maintain brain tissue banks for research. http://www.alzforum.org/dis/dia/bra/default.asp

National Cell Repository for Alzheimer's Disease. Collects information and genetic samples (from those with and without Alzheimer's disease in the family) looking for genetic information that increases the risk of late-life Alzheimer's. www.ncrad.org or http://ncrad.iu.edu/Participate/index.asp

U.S. Government Information on Organ and Tissue Donation and Transplantation. More than 112,000 people are waiting for an organ donation, and the age of the donor is not usually an issue. There are no age limitations on who can donate: whether an organ is eligible for donation depends on the person's physical condition, not age. Newborns as well as senior citizens have been organ donors. http://organdonor.gov/

Judith Horstman is an award-winning journalist who has been a Washington news correspondent, a journalism professor, a Fulbright Scholar, and the recipient of a Knight Science Journalism Fellowship at MIT. Her work has appeared in hundreds of publications worldwide and on the Internet.

This is her fourth brain book in collaboration with *Scientific American* and Jossey-Bass in a series that includes *The* Scientific American *Day in the Life of Your Brain*, *The* Scientific American *Brave New Brain*, and *The* Scientific American *Book of Love, Sex, and the Brain*. Visit her Web site at www.judithhorstman.com.

About Scientific American

Scientific American is at the heart of Nature Publishing Group's consumer media division, meeting the needs of the general public. Founded in 1845, *Scientific American* is the oldest continuously published magazine in the United States and the leading authoritative publication for science in the general media. Together with scientificamerican.com and fourteen local language editions around the world, it reaches more than 5 million consumers and scientists. Other titles include *Scientific American Mind* and *Spektrum der Wissenschaft* in Germany.

A

Acetylcholine, 31, 83, 101, 107

Acetylcholinesterase enzyme, 101

Acetylcholinesterase inhibitors: Alzheimer's treatment using, 100–101; donepezil (Aricept), 100; galantamine (Nivalin, Razadyne), 100

ACTIVE clinical trial, 140, 143

Activities of daily living, 128

Adams, John, 135

Adenauer, Konrad, 15

Adrenalin (or epinephrine), 31

Aerobic exercise: benefits of dance or, 129; swimming and aquatic, 128

Age differences: how the brain changes during, 23; multitasking ability and, 39, 55–57; rates of depression and, 10–12; research on marital status, sexual satisfaction, and, 17–18; self-reported happiness and, 13; on self-reported stress and anger, 14; stroke risk and, 70; study showing exercise benefits at any age, 127–131

Age-related hearing loss, 160

Aging: creativity and, 9; emotional difficulty of dealing with, 195–196; emotional well-being correspondence to, 9, 11–14; hearing loss due to, 160; One Hundred Club of, 20; stroke risk increasing with, 70; studies on sexual desire and aging, 12–13; the usual effects of, 39–40; visual performance decline due to, 143. *See also* Death; Old age

Aging brain: building cognitive reserve in the, 175–184; continuing plasticity of the, 54–55; delaying onset of dementia in the, 11, 32–33; five benefits of orgasms for the, 18; futurists' predicted aids for the, 189–190; the healthy, 39–57; loss of connectivity in the, 45–47; multitasking challenges for the, 39, 55–57; overview of what to expect in the, 37–38; power of meditation for the, 178–180; preparation for living with an, 196–197; the prescription for maintaining a healthy, 193–194; research on the, 3, 5–6; slowing down process but adaptations of the, 51–55; socializing benefits to the, 71, 145, 167–174; threats to your, 62–63; when to address serious symptoms, 64–67. *See also* The brain; Brain development/changes; Brain health

Albert Einstein College of Medicine, 20

Alberts, Jay L., 75

Alcohol: Alzheimer's mistaken for effects of, 68; health benefits of moderate intakes of, 155, 157, 158, 159, 194; reduced to prevent fall injuries, 132

Alcoholism, 68

Alkadhi, Karim, 95

Allergy medications, 85

Allstate-Posit Science study, 144

Alpha-linolenic acid (ALA), 154, 155

Alpha lipoic acid, 160

Alternative therapies, 120–121

Alzheimer, Alois, 90

Alzheimer and Dementia Center
(Methodist Neurological Institute), 164
Alzheimer Disease Neuroimaging
Initiative, 104
Alzheimer Research Forum, 120
Alzheimer's and Dementia (journal), 140
Alzheimer's Association 2011 International
Conference, 69, 106
Alzheimer's disease: benefits of music to
people with, 177–178; bilingual versus
monolingual brains and symptoms of,
138, 139, 142; chronic illness and onset
of, 68, 93, 120; connections between
stress and, 93, 94–96; death rate and
financial burden of, 109; description and
symptoms of, 42, 43–44, 62, 88–89;
diabetes and insulin levels implicated in,
40, 75, 76–77, 80, 93; distinguishing
normal forgetfulness from, 64–67;
emotional and financial costs of, 87–88;
facts about, 90; familial, 91–92, 98, 101,
103–104, 116–117; futurists' predictions
on future of, 189–190, 191; how mental
activity and education delay onset of,
32–33, 137–138; lifestyle relationship to,
11, 88, 93, 98, 104, 114–116; MIC (mild
cognitive impairment) development
into, 69, 89, 96, 106; NIH panel's
determination on lack of prevention for,
113–114. *See also* Dementia; Memory
loss
Alzheimer's disease causes: accumulation
of proteins in the brain, 91–92;
autophagy ("self-eating") breakdown,
97–99; chronic illness connected to, 68,
93, 120; genetic factors as, 91–92, 93, 98,
101, 103–104; lifestyle prevention
approach to understanding, 113–119
Alzheimer's Disease Genetics Study, 92
Alzheimer's Disease International 2011
"World Alzheimer Report," 87, 114
Alzheimer's disease lifestyle prevention:
CFIT (Cognitive Fitness and Innovative
Therapies) practicing, 116–119;

marijuana (THC) used for, 106–108;
NIH report on rejecting, 113–114;
observational studies on, 115–116;
physical exercise for, 47, 124, 126–134;
strategies for optimal brain function,
119–121; UCSF's mathematical model
on, 114–115. *See also* Lifestyle
Alzheimer's disease research: advances and
continued investment in, 109–110;
autophagy breakdown contributing to
onset, 97–99; on benefits of increasing
life space of homebound, 17; on benefits
of moderate intake of alcohol, 158; on
caffeine levels, 162; on how cognitive
reserve protects the brain, 176–184; on
how socializing impacts Alzheimer's,
171, 172; on importance of overall
health, 120; on lifestyle prevention
approach, 113–119; on mitochondria
function linked to synaptic problems,
104–105; on possible causes of, 88,
91–92, 104–106; on possible treatment
or cure, 100–106, 109–110; on risk for
Alzheimer's disease, 98–99; on stress
and Alzheimer's disease, 93, 94–96;
tracking Alzheimer's-specific
biomarkers, 103. *See also* Brain research
Alzheimer's disease risk factors: diabetes
and insulin levels, 40, 75, 76–77, 80, 93;
genetic-related, 91–92, 93, 98, 101,
103–104; heart disease, 40, 93; lifestyle
as, 11, 88, 93, 98, 104, 114–116; obesity
as, 151; research findings on, 98–99;
stress and anxiety, 93, 94–96. *See also*
Chronic illnesses
Alzheimer's disease treatment: alternative
therapies used for, 120–121; FDA
approved medications for, 100–101;
flavonoids shown to help with, 161;
listening to music, 177–178; marijuana
(THC) used for, 106–108; prevention
approach to, 101, 103–104; promising
medication therapies, 102–103, 105–
106; the search for an effective, 100

Alzheimer's Prevention Initiative, 101, 103

American Association for Retired Persons (AARP) studies: on safe sex practices, 19; on satisfaction with sexual activity, 18; Sex, Romance, and Relationships: 2009 AARP Survey of Midlife and Older Adults, 17

Amino acids, 150, 164

Amitriptyline (Elavil), 85

Amnesia, 50

Amnestic mild cognitive impairment (aMCI), 106

Amygdala: brain anatomy and function of, 25; how music depresses activity in the, 177; impact of orgasm on the, 18

Amyloid precursor protein, 91

Anatomy Gifts Registry, 198

Anti-tau compounds, 103

Anticholinergics, 85

Antidepressants, 85

Antioxidants: flavonoids as, 155–159, 161–162; slowing down hearing loss through, 160

Antipsychotics, 85

Anxiety: connections between Alzheimer's disease and, 93, 94–96; exercise to relieve, 124; how music can relieve, 177–178; meditation used to reduce, 178–180; mistaken for dementia, 68; omega-3 oils to relieve, 154. *See also* Stress

ApoE2 gene, 91

ApoE3 gene, 91

ApoE4 gene, 91

Apoliprotein E (Apoe) gene, 91

Aquatic aerobics, 128

Aricept, 100

Arkin, Sharon, 172

Arthritis, 41

Artistic practices, 120

Arts activities study, 176–177

Ashkenazi Jewish elderly people study, 20

Asthma medication, 85

Attitude: building cognitive reserve through positive, 182–184; keeping your brain healthy through positive, 120

Autism, 28

Autism Center of Excellence (UCSD), 28

Autoimmune disorders, 41

Autophagy: Alzheimer's disease linked to breakdown in, 97, 99; description of, 97

Axons, 27

B

B vitamin deficiencies, 164

Bak protein, 160

Balance improvement, 131–134

Ball, Karlene, 136

Banner Sun Health Research Institute, 198

Bardsley, Brent, 198

Barzilai, Nir, 20

Basak, Chandramallika, 137

Bavelier, Daphne, 143

Benadryl, 85

Bennett, Tony, 14

Berries, 155, 156, 157, 159

Beta-amyloid, 76

Beta-amyloid plaque: Alzheimer's connected to, 91, 103; imaging scans showing brain damage due to, 138; mitochrondria function and synaptic problems due to, 104–105; promising therapies to breakdown or prevent, 102–103, 105–106; research on liver as source of, 105; supplements shown to reduce, 163

Beta-amyloid protein: Alzheimer's connected to build-up of, 91, 103; treating Alzheimer's with inhibitors and blockers of, 102–103

Bialystok, Ellen, 138

Biking exercise, 129, 194

Bilingual brains, 138, 139, 142

Blood glucose. *See* Glucose levels

Blood pressure, 123, 171

Blueberries, 155, 156, 157, 159

Boston University of School of Medicine, 78

Botox injections study, 181–182

The brain: Alzheimer's disease linked to autophagy breakdown in, 97, 99; autism symptoms related to big, 28; building cognitive reserve to protect, 175–184; chemistry and electricity of, 31; comparing bilingual and monolingual, 138, 139, 142; connectivity of, 45–47, 104–105; donations of your organs and, 198; executive function of, 30, 125, 136–137; facts about your amazing, 22–23; surges just before death, 199–200. *See also* Aging brain; Neurons; Neurotransmitters

Brain anatomy: amygdala, 18, 25, 77; caudate nucleus, 25; cerebellum, 177; cerebrum ("thinking brain"), 25–26; corpus callosum, 24, 177; differences in musicians and nonmusicians, 177; frontal lobes, 19, 25, 32, 39, 51–52, 143–144; gray matter, 26–27; hindbrain (primitive brain), 24; hippocampus, 25, 48, 126–127, 152, 153, 161, 180; hypothalamus, 25; inferior temporal gyrus, 180; limbic system ("emotional brain"), 24–25; medial temporal lobe, 126; motor cortex, 177; occipital lobe, 25, 143; orbito-frontal cortex, 180; parietal lobes, 25–26; pleasure center (or reward circuit), 25; prefrontal cortex, 25, 47–48, 51–52, 179; right and left hemispheres of the, 24, 56–57; right anterior insula, 179; temporal lobes, 25, 32; thalamus, 180; VTA (ventral tegmental area), 25; white matter, 26–27, 39, 45–47

Brain-derived neurotrophic factor (BDNF), 127

Brain development/changes: during childhood, 28–29; fetal brain, 22, 23–24; the teen brain, 29–30, 32; during the twenties to sixties, 33–35. *See also* Aging brain

Brain donations, 198

Brain Fitness Program (Posit Science), 141

Brain fitness workouts: cognitive training for, 136–145; computer training to keep you driving longer, 143–144; learning a language, 120, 138, 139, 142, 193; research on benefits of, 135–137; strategies for giving yourself, 142, 144–145; testing used to boost learning, 138–139

"Brain foods," 148–149

Brain health: education impact on, 32–33, 137–138; exercise benefits for, 47, 71, 119, 124–134, 194; happy and active lifestyle benefits for, 20, 194; heart-brain connection to, 125–126; how cognitive reserve protects, 175–184; mental activity and stimulation, 32–33, 120; nutrition role in, 120, 147–165, 194; the prescription for maintaining, 193–194; research on brain "workouts" for, 135–137; socializing for, 71, 120, 145, 167–174. *See also* Aging brain; Optimal brain function

Brain injuries: adaptation following, 23; aging and impact of past, 39; cognitive impairment due to past, 63; falling and, 131–132; how the brain heals from, 42

Brain-machine interface, 189

Brain overgrowth, 28

Brain research: ACTIVE clinical trial, 140, 143; on the aging brain, 3, 5–6; amazing facts about the brain learned from, 22–23; on benefits of meditation, 178–180; on benefits of moderate intake of alcohol, 158; on benefits of socializing, 120, 145, 167–172; on benefits of traveling, 178; on Botox injections, frowning, and emotions, 181–182; brain myths disproved by, 49–51; on brain "workouts" to improve cognition, 135–137; on "chemo brain" effects, 81; on cognitive training, 136–145; comparing bilingual and monolingual, 138, 139, 142; distraction exercise, 53; on flavonoids and brain health, 155–159, 161–162; on fructose effects, 153; future development and products from, 187–190; gorilla suit memory study, 49, 51; on healing touch to help stroke recovery, 72–74; on how mitochondria is linked to synaptic problems, 104–105; on how the brain changes through the life span, 21–22; on insulin levels and Alzheimer's disease, 76–77; Language Across the Life Span Project, 54; on marijuana's effects on neurons, 106–108; on mental activity delaying dementia, 32–33, 120; on positive effects of cognitive reserve, 176–184; Seattle Longitudinal Study (1956) on brain changes over life span, 34; on sexual activities and the aging brain, 12–13, 16–19; showing exercise benefits at any age, 127–131; study on walking exercise and improved memory, 126–127; tools used in, 5; on vitamin D deficiency and cognitive function, 165. *See also* Alzheimer's disease research

Brain scan techniques: CAT (computed axial tomography), 4; DTI (diffusion tensor imaging), 5, 46; EEG (electroencephalograph), 4; fMRI (functional magnetic resonance imaging), 4, 46, 51–52, 56, 192–193; MEG (magnetoencephalography), 4; MRI (magnetic resonance imaging), 4, 47–48, 53–54, 179–180; PET (positron emission tomography), 4, 141; SPECT (single photon emission computed tomography), 5

Brain scans: a word of caution about, 5; the aging brain on, 39; as brain research tool, 6; of brains of autistic children, 28;

measuring connectivity in the, 46; Pittsburgh compound B showing brain damage in, 138; tools used for, 4–6

Brain surgery, 189

Brain tumor, 68

Brigham Young University, 168

Brown University, 76, 140

Browne, Brian, 198

Buckner, Randy, 46

Burke, Deborah, 52

C

Cacioppo, John, 170

Caffeine, 148, 158, 162–163

Cajal Institute (Madrid), 108

Calcium, 149, 164

California Institute for Regenerative Medicine (San Francisco), 191

Calment, Jeanne, 20, 158

Campbell, Veronica, 107

Cancer patients, 63, 81

Carbohydrates, 147, 148, 150, 151

Cardiovascular Heart Study, 128

Carstensen, Laura, 12

Casals, Pablo, 15

CAT (computed axial tomography), 4

Caudate nucleus, 25

Ceballos, Maria de, 108

Center for the Study of Traumatic Encephalopathy (Boston University School of Medicine), 78

Centers of Disease Control and Prevention, 19, 78, 79, 131

Cerebellum, 177

Cerebrospinal fluid (CSF), 89

Cerebrum ("thinking brain"), 25–26

Ceroid, 99

CETP gene, 20

Chabris, Christopher, 49, 50–51

Chawla, Lakhmir, 199–200

Chemotherapy ("chemo brain"), 63, 81

Childhood brain development, 28–29

Childhood memories, 44–45

Children with autism, 28

Chlorpheniramine (Chlortrimeton), 85

Chocolate, 155, 156, 157–158, 159, 194

Cholesterol: cognition effects of medications for, 82–83, 84; dark chocolate raising "good," 157; description and function of, 84; exercise to lower, 123; HDL and LDL types of, 76, 157

Christie, Agatha, 15

Chronic illnesses: cognitive impairment due to, 63; diabetes, 40, 63, 69, 93, 123, 124; heart disease, 40, 93, 123, 124, 125–126, 128–130, 171; how physical exercise can prevent and relieve, 123–124; Huntington's disease, 97, 98, 191; Parkinson's disease, 40, 42, 62, 74–75, 96, 133, 187, 190. *See also* Alzheimer's disease risk factors

Churchill, Winston, 72

Cimetidine (Tagamet), 85

Clark, Dick, 72

Clozapine, 85

Coenzyme Q10, 160

Coffee, 162–163, 194

Cognition. *See* Mental abilities

Cognitive Fitness and Innovative Therapies (CFIT), 116–119

Cognitive impairment: "chemo brain" and, 63, 81; correlation between white matter loss and, 46–47; how exercise and healthy activities improve, 10, 42, 47, 71, 75, 119, 123–134; MCI (mild cognitive impairment) form of, 62, 66, 69–70, 80; medications which may cause, 82–85; related to vitamin deficiencies, 68, 121, 164–165; studies on how being homebound increases rate of, 178. *See also* Memory; Mental decline

Cognitive Neurology and Alzheimer's Disease Center (Northwestern University), 53

Cognitive reserve: how attitudes and optimism build, 182–184; how traveling and getting out builds, 178; leisure and creative activities providing, 175, 176–178; power of meditation for building, 178–180; resilience for protecting the brain provided by, 175; smiling and positive emotions to build, 181–182; studies on increased brain function through, 176. *See also* Emotional well-being

Cognitive training: ACTIVE clinical trial on, 140, 143; focusing on executive function, 136–137; growth of businesses engaged in, 139–140; to improve senior driving, 143–144; research on effects on seniors, 136; studies on effectiveness of, 140–144

Cold medications, 85

Cole, Steven, 168

Collines, Michael A., 158

Columbia University, 48, 152

Columbia University Medical Center, 104

Complex carbohydrates, 148, 152

Concussions, 78

Connectivity: aging and loss of, 45–47; of the brain, 46–47; mitochondria function related to synaptic, 104–105

Corpus callosum, 24, 177

Corticosterone, 95

Cortisol hormone, 94–95, 162, 177

Coumadin (Warfarin), 85

Courchesne, Eric, 28

Court sports exercise, 129

Cox, Daniel J., 150

Creativity: creating cognitive reserve by engaging in, 175, 176–178; how traveling and getting out stimulates, 178; keeping your brain healthy through, 120

Cross-country skiing, 129

CT (computed tomography), description of, 4

Cyclosporin D, 105

D

Dalai Lama, 179

Dalì, Salvador, 75

Dance exercise class, 129

Dark chocolate, 155, 156, 157–158, 159, 194

Darwin, Charles, 181

DBS (deep brain stimulation), 74

De la Monte, Suzanne, 76

De Leon, Mony, 152

Death: brain surges just before, 199–200; donating your organs and brain after, 198; emotional reactions to, 195–196; process of dying and, 197, 199. *See also* Aging

Declarative (or explicit) memory, 43

Dehydration, 68

Dementia: B vitamin deficiencies mimicking, 164; chronic illness leading to onset of, 68, 93, 120; conditions which mimic, 68; death rate and financial burden of, 109; diabetes linked to, 40, 75, 76–77, 80, 93; how mental activity and education delay onset of, 32–33, 137–138; lifestyle changes that reduce risk of, 11, 88, 93, 98, 104, 114–116; memory loss due to, 42, 43–44; MIC (mild cognitive impairment) development into, 69, 89, 96, 106; physical exercise for delaying onset of, 47, 124, 126–134; recognizing normal forgetfulness from, 64–67; types and symptoms of, 67–68. *See also* Alzheimer's disease; Memory loss; Mental decline

Dementia with Lewy bodies, 67

Dentate gyrus, 33

Depression: age differences and rates of, 10, 11; Alzheimer's disease linked to, 93; as contributor to MCI, 80; deep brain stimulation to treat, 42; description of, 63; impact on health by, 184; medications for, 85; mistaken for dementia, 68, 79; in older people, 78–80; overmedicating due to, 79; physical exercise to help, 123; signs that treatment is needed for, 80

Desyryl, 85

Diabetes: accelerating MCI progression to dementia, 69; Alzheimer's and dementia linked to, 40, 75, 76–77, 80, 93; description of, 63; exercise benefits for, 123, 124; Parkinson's disease linked to, 75, 77. *See also* Glucose levels; Type 2 diabetes

Diet. *See* Foods; Nutrition

Digoxin, 85

Diphenhydramine (Benadryl), 85

Disney films, 12

Distraction exercise, 53

DNA (deoxyribonucleic acid), 34, 92

Docosahexaenoic acid (DHA), 154, 155

Donating your brain, 198

Donepezil (Aricept), 100

Dopamine: function of, 31; Parkinson's disease and degeneration of, 74, 75; Parkinson's disease–like conditions brought on by, 96; study on brain training software impact on, 141

Douglas, Kirk, 72

Driving safety study, 16

Driving skills study, 143–144

Drug interactions, 68

DTI (diffusion tensor imaging): description of, 5; measuring loss of connectivity of the brain, 46

Dylan, Bob, 14

E

Earhart, Gammon M., 134

Edison, Thomas Alva, 16

Educated brains: increased brain health longevity of, 137–138; rapid development of dementia after onset, 32–33. *See also* Learning

EEG (electroencephalograph), 4

Eicosapentaenoic acid (EPA), 154

Einstein, Albert, 16

Elavil, 85

Elder statesman, 9

Electra (Sophocles), 15

Electroencephalography, 4

Emotional well-being: how aging increases, 9, 10, 12–14; how meditation can provide, 178–180. *See also* Cognitive reserve

Emotions: areas of the brain that regulate, 180; Botox injections study on frowning and, 181–182; how emotional responses influence our feelings, 181–182; how meditation helps to regulate, 178–180; how music soothes the, 177–178; related to aging and death, 195–196

Endorphins, 31

Epigenome, 34

Epilepsy seizures, 42

Epinephrine (or adrenaline), 31

Erectile dysfunction, 18–19

Ersner-Hersfield, Hal, 192

Estrogen, 41

Executive function: aerobic exercise and improved, 125; cognitive training focusing on, 136–137; processes allowed by, 30

Exercise. *See* Physical exercise/activity

Experiences: ability of older brain to tap into, 51; gorilla suit study on memory of unexpected, 49, 51; how long-term memories are created from, 43, 48, 50; how the short-term memory functions with new, 43, 48; TOT (tip-of-the-tongue), 52. *See also* Memories

Explicit (or declarative) memory, 43

Eyewitness testimony: hypnosis and unreliable, 49–50; remembering phenomenon and, 50

F

Fall injuries: exercise to prevent seniors from, 131–134; "fear-of-falling gait" and, 133; as most common cause of brain injuries in seniors, 131; TBI (traumatic brain injury), 77–78

Falstaff (Verdi), 15

Familial Alzheimer's: Alzheimer's Prevention Initiative clinical trials on, 101, 103; amyloid precursor protein on chromosome 21 related to, 91–92; Casa Neurosciencias clinic treating, 116–117; Columbian families suffering from, 116–117; severity of onset of, 98

The Fantastic Voyage (film), 189

"Fear-of-falling gait," 133

Fetal brain: development of the, 23–24; neurons and neuron pruning in the, 22

Fields, R. Douglas, 44

Fight-or-flight response, 18

Fish oil, 150, 154–155

Flavonoids: description of, 155; health benefits of, 155–159, 161–162; subgroups of, 156

fMRI (functional magnetic resonance imaging): comparing young and old brains during mental activities, 51–52; description of, 5; measuring brain activity when thinking of our future self, 192–193; measuring loss of connectivity in the brain, 46; measuring multitasking ability, 56

Folic acid, 164

Foods: alcohol, 68, 132, 158; "brain," 148–149; fructose-rich, 152–153; glucose-rich, 153; rich in flavonoids, 155–159, 161–162; rich in omega-3 fatty acids, 150, 154–155; water intake, 161–162. *See also* Nutrition

Forgetfulness: description of minor incidents of, 64; recognizing serious cognitive problems with, 64–67

Fox, Michael J., 74

Franklin, Benjamin, 15

Free radicals, 160

Friendships: developed in later life, 173–174; mental health related to our, 170–171; physical health benefits of, 171

Frontal lobes: brain anatomy and, 25; driving skills related to, 143–144; recall

function of, 32; seniors' ability to
activate, 39, 51–52
Frontotemporal dementia, 68
Frostig, Ron, 72, 73–74
Fructose, 152–153
Furosemide, 85
Future-self thinking, 192–193

G
GABA (gamma-aminobutyric acid), 31
Galantamine (Nivalin, Razadyne), 100
Gallagher, Michela, 52
Gallup survey on negative memories
(2008), 13
Garner, James, 72
Gazzaley, Adam, 55, 56
Gender differences: dementia and
Alzheimer's disease rates and, 40–41; in
disease patterns, 41; in the healthy aging
brain, 40–41; life expectancy and, 40;
sexual dysfunction and, 18–19. *See also*
Men; Women
Genetic factors: Alzheimer's disease linked
to, 93; research findings on Alzheimer's
risk and, 91–92, 98, 101, 103; research
tracking Alzheimer's-specific
biomarkers, 103
Genital warts, 19
Genome, 34
George Washington University Medical
Center, 199
Georgia State University, 153
Gerdner, Linda A., 177
Geriatric depression Scale, 177
Ginkgo biloba, 120–121, 163
Gitelman, Darren, 54
Glial cells, 26
Glucose: natural food sources of, 153;
optimal for brain health, 148, 150
Glucose levels: Alzheimer's and dementia
linked to high, 40, 75, 76–77, 80, 93;
"senior moments" and, 151–152; tai chi
connected to lowering, 132. *See also*
Diabetes; Nutrition

Glutamate, 31
Gonorrhea, 19
Gorilla suit memory study, 49, 51
Graham, Billy, 75
Graveline, Duane, 82, 83
Gray matter, 26–27
Great late achievers: honor roll of
examples of, 15–16; research on
accomplishments of, 14
Green, Shawn, 143
Guggenheim Museum (NYC), 15
Guillaume, Robert, 72

H
Hackney, Madeleine E., 134
Happiness: age differences and self-
reported, 13; brain health and lifestyle
of, 20, 194; how aging increases, 9, 10,
12–14; longevity connected to, 171;
marital, 17
Harvard School of Public Health, 168
Harvard University, 81
HDL cholesterol, 76, 157
Head injuries: concussions, 78; falls and,
77–78; impairment due to past, 63; TBI
(traumatic brain injury), 63, 77–78
Healing touch, 72–74
Health and Retirement Study report
(2008), 169
Healthy activities, aging myths related to,
10
The healthy aging brain: connectivity of,
46–47; continuing plasticity of the,
54–55; gender differences in the, 40–41;
how the memory works in the, 41–45;
multitasking and the, 39, 55–57;
multitasking by, 55–57; slower pace but
adaptations of, 51–55; TOT (tip-of-the-
tongue) experiences and, 52; the usual
effects of aging on, 39–40; white matter
importance to, 45–46
Healthy Aging (Weil), 137
Hearing loss, 160
Heart-brain connection, 125–126

Heart disease: Alzheimer's disease and dementia linked to, 40, 93; exercise to prevent, 123, 124; how socializing improves, 171; study on walking exercise benefits for, 128–129
Hemoglobin levels, 120
Hemorrhagic stroke, 70, 72
Hess, Thomas M., 183
High blood pressure, 123, 171
High-fructose corn syrup, 153
Hindbrain (primitive brain), 24
Hippocampus: aging impact on volume of, 126; effects of blood glucose in the, 152; flavonoids spurring growth of new cells in, 161; how meditation affects the, 180; memory role of the, 48; neuron production in the, 25; study on insulin resistance impact on, 153; study on walking exercise impact on, 126–127
HIV/AIDS, 19
Holt-Lunstad, Julianne, 168, 169
Homocysteine, 164
Huntington's disease, 97, 99, 191
Hypnosis-induced recollection, 49–50
Hypothalamus, 25

I
IGF-1 receptor, 77
Illoila, Fiji Josefa, 75
Imatinib, 105–106
Imipramine (Tofranil), 85
Implicit (or nondeclarative) memory, 43–44
Inferior temporal gyrus, 180
Inflammation: dangers of systemic, 120; how socializing lowers, 171; omega-3 oils to relieve, 154
Insight Meditation, 179
InSight program, 144
Institut National de la Santé et de la Recherche Médicale (France), 157
Insulin: Alzheimer's disease and levels of, 40, 75, 76–77, 80, 93; Parkinson's disease and levels of, 75, 77
Internet friends, 173–174

Interview research tool, 5
The Invisible Gorilla (Chabris and Simons), 51
Iron nutrient, 148
Iron supplement, 163–164
Ischemic stroke, 70, 72

J
Jagger, Mick, 14
James, Bryan, 178
James, P. D., 15
James, William, 181
John Paul II, Pope, 75
Johns Hopkins University, 52, 106
Journal of Alzheimer's Disease, 162
Journal of Neuroscience, 28
Journal of Pain, 182
Journal of the American Geriatrics Society, 79

K
Kael, Pauline, 75
Kaiser Permanente Foundation Research Institute (Oakland), 151, 169
Kandel, Eric, 16
Karolinska Institute (Sweden), 131, 141
Keller, Helen, 15
Kemper, Susan, 54
Kent State University, 139
Kirtan Kriya meditation, 180
Knutson, Brian, 192
Kosik, Kenneth S., 116–117
Kurlan, Roger, 133

L
Laboratory tests, 6
LaFerla, Frank M., 190
Language Across the Life Span Project, 54
Language learning, 120, 138, 139, 142, 193
Lasix (furosemide), 85
LDL cholesterol, 76, 157
Learning: the aging brain and, 11; aging loss of myelin affecting ability for new, 45–46; changes in white matter and neurons when, 27; how it delays onset

of dementia, 32–33, 137–138; a language, 120, 138, 139, 142, 193; studies on how testing boosts, 138–139. *See also* Educated brains

Left brain hemisphere: description of, 24; multitasking role of the, 56–57

Letenneur, Luc, 157

Levetiracetam, 106

Lewis, Michael, 182

Life expectancy: gender differences in, 40; happiness connected to longevity, 171; historic increases in, 1–2; positive attitudes connected to longevity, 183–184

Life span: how autophagy may determine, 99; Seattle Longitudinal Study (1956) on brain changes over, 34; trend toward lengthened, 196

Lifestyle: lowering risk for type 2 diabetes, 77; reducing stroke risk with changes in, 72; role in health of your brain by, 20, 194; strategies for optimal brain function, 119–121. *See also* Alzheimer's disease lifestyle prevention; Physical exercise/activity

Limbic system ("emotional brain"), 24–25

Lipitor, 82, 102

Lipofuscin, 97, 99

Liquids (nutrient), 148

Lithium, 106

Living will, 197

Llewellyn, David, 165

Loneliness, 170

Loneliness Scale, 177

Long-term memory: amnesia sufferers and impaired, 50; description of, 43; how it functions to retain memories, 48

Lou Gehrig's disease, 172

Loyola University Chicago Stritch School of Medicine, 158

Lustig, Cindy, 51

M

Macready, Anna, 159

Malleret, Gaël, 48

Marijuana (THC): negative effects on young neurons by, 106–107; positive effects on neurons in adults with Alzheimer's, 107–108

Marital happiness, 17

Marketwatch cognitive training report, 140

Mayo Clinic study of aging (2010), 41

Mayo Clinic's Brain Fitness Program study, 141

Medial temporal lobe, 126

Medical power of attorney, 197

Medications: acetylcholinesterase inhibitors, 100–101; anti-tau compounds, 103; anticholinergics, 85; antidepressants, 85; beta-amyloid aggregation blockers, 102; beta-amyloid inhibitors, 102; cholesterol-lowering statins, 82–83, 84; cognitive impairment due to, 63, 82–85; cyclosporin D, 105; FDA approved Alzheimer's disease, 100–101; imatinib, 105–106; levetiracetam, 106; Lipitor, 102; lithium, 106; medical marijuana (THC), 106–108; neuroprotective agents, 103; NMDA (*N*-methyl-*D*-aspartate) receptor antagonist, 101; promising therapies for Alzheimer's disease, 102–103, 105–106; Prozac, 102; reduced to prevent fall injuries, 132; vaccines that clear beta-amyloid, 102

Meditation, 178–180

MedWatch, 83, 84

MEG (magnetoencephalography), 4

Meir, Golda, 15

Memantine (Namenda), 101

Memento (film), 50

Memories: aging and recollection of negative versus positive, 13–14; created when messages are sent across synapses, 43; forgetting role in remembering, 47–48; how brain chemistry affects, 43; how phobias are created by childhood, 44–45; how repetition creates, 44; how the aging brain adapts to access, 53–55. *See also* Experiences

Memory: cognitive impairment of, 11; five myths about, 48–51; gorilla suit study on, 49, 51; how it works, 41–45; importance of our, 41–42; long-term, 43, 48, 50; MRI measuring work pair, 47–48; short-term (working), 43, 48; TOT (tip-of-the-tongue) experiences and, 52. *See also* Cognitive impairment

Memory loss: aMCI (amnestic mild cognitive impairment) contribution to, 106; "chemo brain" and, 63, 81; cholesterol-lowering statins and, 82–83, 84; cognitive impairment and, 11; correlation between white matter loss and, 46–47; future development for preventing and reversing, 190–191; how foods rich in flavonoids improve, 155–159, 161–162; neurological and psychiatric conditions causing, 65; "senior moments," 151–152; study on walking exercise and improved, 126–127; symptoms of serious, 64–67; why the better educated with dementia rapidly suffer, 32–33. *See also* Alzheimer's disease; Dementia

Memory myths: amnesia sufferers cannot remember their name, 50; hypnosis can improve memory, 49–50; memories are forever, 50; of memory as passively recorded, 49; unexpected occurrence is likely to be noticed, 49

Men: dementia and Alzheimer's disease rates among, 40–41; impact of age on sexual activities in, 18–19. *See also* Gender differences

Mental abilities: brain connectivity and, 45–47; brain fitness products to improve, 139–142, 144–145; changes between 20s and 60s, 33–35; comparing bilingual and monolingual brains, 138, 139, 142; computer training to improve driving-related, 143–144; glucose levels and, 148, 150; how foods rich in flavonoids improve, 155–159, 161–162;

mental activity and stimulation to maintain, 32–33, 120; research on "workouts" to improve, 135–137; strategies for optimal brain function, 119–121

Mental decline: "chemo brain" and, 81; coming to grips with slippage, 71; depression and, 78–80; how diabetes may impact, 75–77; how medications can impact, 82–85; Parkinson's disease and, 40, 42, 74–75; signs of, 66; stroke impact on, 70, 72–74; studies on how being homebound increases rate of, 178; summary of common things resulting in, 62–63; symptoms of serious, 64–67; TBI (traumatic brain injury) and, 77–78. *See also* Cognitive impairment; Dementia

Mental health: counseling or therapy to improve, 71; how relationships impact our, 170–171; how socializing can improve, 71, 120, 145, 167–174; loneliness and isolation impact on, 170

Mental stimulation, 119–120

Methionine, 149

Methodist Neurological Institute (Houston), 164

Metz, Gerlinde A. S., 96

Michaels, Brett, 72

Michelangelo, 15

Middle-aged brain, 34

Mild cognitive impairment (MCI): aMCI (amnestic mild cognitive impairment) form of, 106; depression as contributor to, 80; description and symptoms of, 62, 66; progression to Alzheimer's or dementia, 69–70, 89, 96

Milner, Brenda, 16

Mindfulness Meditation, 179, 180

Minerals, 150

Mitochondria function, 104–105

Monje, Michelle L., 81

Monolingual versus bilingual brains, 138, 139, 142

Moses, Anna Mary Robertson (Grandma Moses), 15

Mossman, Kaspar, 142

Motor cortex, 177

Motor vehicle crashes study, 16

MRI (magnetic resonance imaging): description of, 4; measuring memory retention of word pairs, 47–48; showing aging brain during mental activities, 53–54; showing differences in practitioners of meditation, 179–180; showing results of walking exercise on hippocampus, 126–127

Muhammad Ali, 74, 75

Multitasking: the aging brain and difficulty with, 39, 55–57; fMRI study on age differences and ability for, 56

Multivitamins, 16

Music: emotional benefits of, 177; self-medicating with, 177–178

Myelin: aging and reduced, 39, 45–46; description of, 26; formation and functions of, 26–27; during the 20s to 60s, 33

N

Namenda, 101

National Cell Repository for Alzheimer's Disease, 92

National Endowment for the Arts, 176

National Institute of Child Health and Human Development, 44

National Institute on Aging, 20, 54, 125, 136

National Institutes of Health (NIH), 104, 109, 113–114, 188

Nature (journal), 143

Neafsey, Edward J., 158

Neal, Patricia, 72

Neurites, 99

Neuroenhancers, 189

Neurofibrillary tangles, 94

Neurogenesis: description of process, 33–34; predictions on future research developments for, 190; studies on exercise benefits for, 81

Neurology (journal), 120

Neuronal networks: aging and slowing down of, 39; plasticity of the aging brain, 54–55

Neurons: the aging brain and, 39; brain anatomy and location of, 26; cortisol effects on, 95; fetal brain, 22, 24; hippocampus production of new, 25, 48; how exercise encourages growth of, 42; how learning creates changes in, 27; loss after birth and during adolescence, 22; marijuana's effects on the, 106–108; neurogenesis and loss of, 33–34, 81, 190; synapses between, 43, 52; during the 20s to 60s, 33–34. *See also* The brain

Neuroplasticity, 34

Neuroprotective agents, 103

Neurotransmitters: acetylcholine, 31, 83, 101, 107; description of, 31; dopamine, 31, 74, 75, 96, 141; endorphins, 31; epinephrine (or adrenaline), 31; functions in the brain, 31; GABA (gamma-aminobutyric acid), 31; glutamate, 31; memory loss related to age-related depletion of, 46–47; oxytocin, 31; Parkinson's disease and degeneration of, 74–75; serotonin, 31. *See also* The brain

New York University, 152

Nivalin, 100

NMDA (*N*-methyl-*D*-aspartate) receptor antagonist, 101

Nogo-A, 45, 46

Nondeclarative (or implicit) memory, 43–44

North Carolina State University, 183

Northwestern University, 53

Nortriptyline (Pamelor), 85

Nurk, Eha, 157

Neurogenesis, 33–34

Nutrition: basic facts about the brain and, 147–151; "brain foods," 148–149; brain health and importance of, 120, 147–165, 194; caffeine, 148, 162–163; flavonoids, 155–159, 161–162; fructose, 152–154; omega-3 fatty acids, 150, 154–155; USDA guidelines on diet and, 161, 165; vitamin supplements and, 121, 163–165. *See also* Foods; Glucose levels

O

Obesity: as Alzheimer's disease risk factor, 151; fructose blamed for increased, 152–153
Observation research tool, 5
Occipital lobe, 25, 143
Oedipus at Colonus (Sophocles), 15
Old age: changes in life expectancy and, 1–2; defining, 2–3; driving safety during, 16; great late achievers during, 14–16; myth of a sad, 10–12; One Hundred Club of, 20. *See also* Aging
Old age myths: list of major, 10–11; media perpetuation of, 12
"Old old age," 3
Olfactory bulb, 33
Omega-3 fatty acids, 150, 154–155
One Hundred Club, 20
Optimal brain function: brain fitness products for, 139–142, 144–145; brain "workouts" for, 135–145; CFIT approach to, 116–119; computer training to keep you driving longer, 143–144; debate over lifestyle preventive approach to, 113–116; strategies for maintaining, 119–121, 144–145. *See also* Aging brain; Brain health
Optimistic attitude: brain health through, 120; building cognitive reserve through, 182–184
Orbito-frontal cortex, 180
Osteoporosis, 41
Otello (Verdi), 15
Overmedication, 68

Oxidation of cells, 160
Oxytocin, 31

P

Pain: how music can relieve, 177–178; how touching can reduce perception of, 171
Pamelor, 85
Parent, Marise B., 153
Parietal lobes, 25–26
Parkinson's disease: demographics of, 62; "fear-of-falling gait" mistaken for, 133; flavonoids shown to help with, 161; futurists' predictions on future of, 190; how stress may hasten onset of, 96; impact on brain areas involving motor control, 42, 62; insulin implications in, 75, 77; mental decline due to, 40, 62, 74–75; new scientific breakthroughs with, 187; vigorous exercise to improve symptoms of, 75
Pediatric (journal), 16
Personal hygiene deficit, 66
PET (positron emission tomography): brain training software studies using, 141; description of, 4
Pets, 174
Phenylalanine, 149, 158
Phobia creation, 44–45
Physical exercise/activity: aging myths related to, 10; brain health benefits of, 47, 71, 119, 124–134, 194; chronic illness relief and prevention through, 123–124; as delaying onset of Alzheimer's and dementia, 47, 124, 126–134; different types of effective, 128–129; how it helps heal brain injuries, 42; impact of walking exercise on the brain, 126–127; to improve balance and prevent falls, 131–134; to improve Parkinson's disease symptoms, 75; improving mental decline through, 71; for improving vision and reaction time, 143; for optimal brain function, 119, 145; stress reduced through, 42;

studies showing benefits at any age, 127–131. *See also* Lifestyle

Physical therapy for stroke recovery, 72

Picasso, Pablo, 15

Pittsburgh compound B, 138

Pleasure center (reward circuit), 25

Pomona College, 52

Posit Science, 141, 144

Positive attitude: building cognitive reserve through, 182–184; keeping your brain healthy through, 120

Positive self-talk, 184

Potassium, 164

Prednisolone, 85

Prefrontal cortex: brain anatomy of, 25; meditation to offset age-related thinning of, 179; MRI measuring memory retention and activity in, 47–48

Presenilin 1 gene, 91

Presenilin 2 gene, 91, 105

Proinflammatory cytokines, 120

Pronin, Emily, 192

Protein (dietary), 150

Proteins: Alzheimer's related to accumulation in brain, 91–92; Bak, 160; beta-amyloid, 91, 102, 103; study on caffeine impact on Alzheimer's and related, 162; tau, 91, 94, 103

Prozac, 102

Pseudoephedrine, 85

Psychological assessment, 66–67

Pyc, Mary, 139

R

Radiation treatment, 81

Ranitidine (Zantac), 85

Rawson, Katherine, 139

Razadyne, 100

Remembering, 50

Reading glasses, 64

Red wine, 155, 157, 159, 194

Reese, Della, 72

Relationships: later life friendships and, 173–174; mental health related to our,

170–171; physical health benefits of, 171

Religious practices: keeping brain healthy through, 120; meditation as, 178–180

Reno, Janet, 75

Resilience. *See* Cognitive reserve

Retirement myths, 10

Reviews of Therapeutics (journal), 84

Reward circuit (pleasure center), 25

Richards, Keith, 14

Richards, Marcus, 130

Right anterior insula, 179

Right brain hemisphere: description of, 24; multitasking role of the, 56–57

Roe, Catherine M., 138

Román, Gustavo C., 164

Rooney, Andy, 15

Rovio, Suvi, 131

Ruan, Hongyu, 172

Rubinstein, Arthur, 15

Rush University Medical Center (Chicago), 96, 137, 169, 178

S

Safe sex practices, 19

Salk Institute for Biological Studies (San Diego), 94, 125, 190

Schumann, Cynthia, 28

Schwab, Martin E., 45

Schweitzer, Albert, 15

Science (journal), 56–57

Scientific American (journal), 44, 140, 142

Seattle Longitudinal Study (1956), 34

Seligman, Martin E. P., 184

Senior driving programs, 144

Senior exercise programs, 71

"Senior moments," 151–152

Serotonin, 31

Sex, Romance, and Relationships: 2009 AARP Survey of Midlife and Older Adults, 17

Sexual activities: impact of age on male, 18–19; physical benefits to the brain, 18

Sexual desire studies, 12–13, 16–19

Sexual satisfaction: benefits of orgasms for the aging brain, 18; research on marital status, age difference, and, 17–18

Sexually transmitted diseases, 19

SharpBrains, 140

Shaw, George Bernard, 171

Short-term (working) memory: description of, 43; how memories are retained using, 48

Simons, Daniel, 49, 50–51

60 Minutes (TV news show), 15

Skype, 174

Small, Scott, 152

Smiling, 181–182

Smoking, 93

Snyder, Peter, 140–141, 144

Socializing: aging and benefits of, 1, 71; description of, 167; finding and making friends in later life, 173–174; for optimal brain function, 120, 145; research studies on benefits of, 167–172

Sod1 gene mutation, 172

Sodium levels, 164

Sophocles, 15

Soy isoflavones, 156, 159

SPECT (single photon emission computed tomography), 5

Spinal tap, 89

Spiritual practices: keeping your brain healthy through, 120; meditation as, 178–180

St. John's wort, 163

Stanford University, 183, 192

Statins, 82–83, 84

Stone, Arthur, 14

Stone, Sharon, 72

Stony Brook University, 14

Stress: aging and self-reported, 14; connections between Alzheimer's disease and, 93, 94–96; cortisol hormone released during, 94–95, 162, 177; how exercise reduces, 42, 124; how music can relieve, 177–178; meditation used to reduce, 178–180; mistaken for dementia, 68; optimal brain function by reducing, 120. *See also* Anxiety

Strittmatter, Stephen M., 45

Stroke: aging as risk of, 70; Alzheimer's disease linked to, 93; brain damage due to, 42; dementia as by-product of, 40; description and process of, 62, 70; healing touch to help recovery from, 72–74; how exercise reduces, 124; lifestyle changes that reduce risk of, 72; medical effects of, 70; prognosis for recovery from, 70, 72; signs of a, 73; yoga therapy following a, 132

Stroke (journal), 73

Suicide rates, 79

Supplements and vitamins, 120–121, 163–165

Swimming exercise, 128, 194

Sylvette (Picasso), 15

Synapses: connecting neurons, 43; cortisol effects on, 95; mitochondria function linked to problems with, 104–105; study on aging brain of rats and, 52

Syphilis, 19

Systemic inflammation, 120

T

Tagamet, 85

Tai chi, 71, 129, 132, 194

Tau protein, 91, 94, 103

Tea, 157, 159, 162, 194

Teacher (Keller), 15

Technical University of Munich (Germany), 182

Temporal lobes: aging impact on, 32; brain anatomy of, 25

Tetrahydrocannabinol (THC) [marijuana]: negative effects on young neurons by, 106–107; positive effects on neurons in adults with Alzheimer's, 107–108

Thalamus, 180

Theobromine, 158

Theophyline, 85

"Thinking brain" (cerebrum), 25–26

Thorazine, 85
Thyroid imbalances, 68
Tinetti, Mary, 78
Tissue plasminogen activator (tPA), 70
Tofu, 155, 156, 157
TOT (tip-of-the-tongue) experiences, 52
Touching therapy, 171
Transcendental meditation, 179
Traumatic brain injury (TBI): description of, 63; falls causing, 77–78
Traveling activities, 178
Trazadone (Desyryl), 85
Tricyclic antidepressants, 85
Trinity College (Dublin), 107
Trofranil, 85
Trombetti, Andrea, 133
Turmeric, 163
Turner, Tina, 14
Twin studies, 20
Type 1 diabetes, 75
Type 2 diabetes, 75, 76–77. *See also* Diabetes
Tyrosine, 149, 150

U
UFOV (useful field of view), 143, 144
Umberson, Debra, 17
Union College, 49
Unitarian Universalists, 173
University College London, 130
University of Alabama at Birmingham, 136
University of Arizona, 172
University of Arkansas for Medical Sciences, 177
University of California, Irvine, 72, 190
University of California, Los Angeles, 168, 180
University of California, San Diego, 28
University of California, San Francisco, 55, 114, 125
University of Cambridge (England), 165
University of Dortmund (Germany), 53
University of Houston, 95

University of Illinois, 49, 137
University of Iowa, 172
University of Lethbridge (Alberta), 96
University of Manchester (England), 165
University of Michigan, Ann Arbor, 51
University of Northumbria, 151
University of Oslo (Norway), 157
University of Pittsburgh, 128
University of Reading (England), 159
University of Rochester, 133, 143
University of Texas at Austin, 17
University of Toronto, 32
University of Virginia Health System, 150
University of Washington, 34, 75
University of Western Australia, 130
University of Zurich, 45
Unsaturated fatty acids, 149
Untreated chronic conditions, 68
U.S. Department of Agriculture (USDA), 161, 165
U.S. Food and Drug Administration, 83, 100
Useful field of view (UFOV), 143, 144

V
Vaccines (clearing beta-amyloid), 102
Vaginitis, 19
Valera, Eamon de, 15
van Praag, Henrietta, 125
Vascular dementia, 67
Ventral tegmental area (VTA), 25
Verdi, Giuseppi, 15
Victoria, Queen (England), 15
Visual performance, 143
Vitamin B_1, 149, 164
Vitamin C, 164
Vitamin D, 68, 78, 132, 164–165
Vitamin deficiencies: cognitive failings related to, 121, 164–165; Vitamin B and D, 68
Vitamin supplements, 121, 163–165
Vitamins: necessary for good health, 150; nutritional requirements for, 150, 163–165

W

Wageningen University (Netherlands), 183

Wagner, Anthony, 48

Walking exercise: "fear-of-falling gait," 133; lowering risks of dementia with, 128; studies showing benefits at any age, 127–131; study on memory improvement due to, 126–127

Warfarin, 85

Washington University, 138

Washington University School of Medicine, 134

Water intake, 161–162

Watson, James, 92

Weill, Andrew, 137

White matter: aging and loss of connectivity provided by, 45–47; aging and reduced, 39; correlation between memory loss and loss of, 46–47; description of, 26–27; the healthy aging brain and, 45–46

Wii (virtual reality sports), 72

Wilkinson, Lucy, 151

Willis, Sherry, 34

Wilson, Robert S., 96, 137

Wine intake, 155, 157, 159, 194

Women: dementia and Alzheimer's disease rates among, 40–41; life expectancy of, 40. *See also* Gender differences

Woodruff, Bob, 42

Working memory. *See* Short-term (working) memory

"World Alzheimer Report" (2011), 87, 114

Wright, Frank Lloyd, 15

Wu, Chun-Fang, 172

Y

Yaffe, Kristine, 125

Yale School of Medicine's Program in Geriatrics, 78, 132

Yan, Shirley ShiDu, 104

Yoga, 71, 129, 132, 194

Z

Zantac, 85

Zen Meditation, 179, 180

Zinc, 149

Zukor, Adolph, 15